What People Are Saying About Shea Vaughn . . .

"I wholeheartedly support the SheaNetics program for people of all ages."

—Dr. Michael E. Kordecki, D.P.T., S.C.S., A.T.C., Principle Owner of
PRAXIS Physical Therapy and Human Performance

"I have been exercising for years but only with Shea's method was I able to achieve the results I wanted. She completely changed my body and made me stronger. Thank you, Shea!"

—Joanna, SheaNetics Student

"My body has changed completely by doing Shea's program! I am the most fit I have been in my life. I feel long, lean, and firm. All of my family and friends tell me how fit and healthy I look and seem."

—Anne, SheaNetics Student

"I practice internal medicine. What I found in SheaNetics was a program that improved my strength, increased my flexibility, and reduced stress."

—Michael Sommerfeld, M.D., Internal Medicine

"Shea Vaughn is amazing! She has been an inspiration to both my wife and me. She completely changed our bodies and our outlook on living healthy and fulfilling our life goals. We believe in the 5 Living Principles and practice them every day."

—Mark, SheaNetics Student

"I think that there is key role in using SheaNetics as a bridge program to get athletes back to full sports with a key role in injury prevention."

—Roger N. Chams, M.D., Orthopedic Surgeon, Sports Medicine
Arthroscopic Reconstructive Knee & Shoulder Surgery
Fellowship, Southern California Orthopedic Institute

"Shea is a dynamic, inspiring, and genuinely compassionate being who is full of life, energy, and love. She is unconditional with her giving nature and can root people on to discover a potential within themselves they didn't know they had. She is truly a life coach who has a great understanding of health, fitness, and life-force energy and how to manifest that in one's life. I have been constantly inspired by her to go beyond perceived limits and am blessed to have her support with me every step of the way. But most important of all, I am grateful to be able to call a person of such great ability, character, and strength, my mother."

—Valeri, Producer

"Shea is an amazing person. She has been a continuous example of strength and resilience to me and many others. She was the first person to ignite my ongoing fire for exercise and good nutrition as they relate to the sports I pursue."

—Danny Ferrone, Personal Trainer and Martial Artist

"My mom has always been ahead of her time in seeking and understanding total and sustainable body fitness, inside and out. I am excited that, with this book, she will be able to reach people throughout the world and bring to them strength and wellness through her program that will give them a life they never knew they could have."

—Victoria, producer

Acknowledgments

My mother Jeanette: who loved me unconditionally, allowed me to be me, and taught me life's important values.

My children: Victoria, Valeri, and Vincent, who are "The Beat of My Heart," precious gifts of love, and my greatest teachers.

My grandchildren: Dexter, Stella, Veronica, Vivianna, and Locklyn, who are the joy of my life, the laughter of my heart, and the hope of our future.

My husband Steve: with an endless amount of love and support, he is the reason my life's accomplishments and visions are realized.

My stepson Danny: who is a special offering of love, a cherished blessing, and a hero and role model to all of us.

My sister Gail and brother Jerry: who give love and support without judgment, are the pillars that sustain us all together, and are the shoulders on which I can always lean.

My niece and nephews: Jeff, Leslie, Daryl, and Bryan; my aunts Georgia and Kathy Jo; and my half sisters and brother Linda, Marion, and Gary; who have enriched my life beyond anything they might imagine.

My family, friends, and students, and to all those who have graced my life and who have inspired and encouraged me by believing in me. This book is because of you! It embraces my passion and invites me to touch the hearts of many and change lives by making healthier choices and setting good examples. My heart is filled with the hopes and dreams that we can all live an enriching and loving life.

SHEA VAUGHN'S

Breakthrough

The 5 Living Principles to Defeat Stress, Look Great & Find Total Well-Being

Shea Vaughn

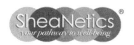

Health Communications, Inc.
Deerfield Beach, Florida

www.hcibooks.com

The information contained in this book is not intended to replace the advice of a physician. All content is provided for information purposes and readers should consult their own physicians concerning any health or exercise program.

Library of Congress Cataloging-in-Publication Data

Vaughn, Shea.
   Shea Vaughn's breakthrough : the 5 living principles to defeat stress, look great, and find total well-being / Shea Vaughn.
      p. cm.
   Includes index.
   ISBN-13: 978-0-7573-1593-0 (trade paper)
   ISBN-10: 0-7573-1593-3 (trade paper)
   ISBN-13: 978-0-7573-9165-1 (e-book)
   1. Women—Psychology.   2. Mind and body.   3. Women--Mental health.   I. Title.
   HQ1206.V38 2011
   155.3'3391—dc23

                                                                            2011027153

Publisher: Health Communications, Inc.
            3201 S.W. 15th Street
            Deerfield Beach, FL 33442-8190

Borris Powell - cover, page 4, and chapter 8 fashion designs
Giuliano Correia - cover, page 4, and chapter 8 sequence photography
Freddie Anaya - cover, page 4, and chapter 8 sequence makeup
Asha Spacek - artistic director
Rod Roberts - photography
Sarah Squire - hair and makeup
Nevena Zee - hair styling
Michele Matrisciani - contributing writer
Cover design by Justin Rockowitz
Interior design and formatting by Lawna Patterson Oldfield

Contents

Foreword

Medicine is an ever-changing industry. Beginning centuries ago with the simplest investigations into the functions of the human body, its practice has evolved into the precise and complex science we know today. In a short time we've seen advances ranging from the invention of penicillin to the mapping of the human genome.

Most recently, medicine has benefited from the internet's ability to fulfill the public's need for information. In turn, the medical community has recognized medicine as a service trade. Many hospitals around the world have taken up the patient-first banner, including the Cancer Treatment Centers of America hospitals, where I have practiced for the past twenty years as a gastroenterologist and nutritionist, along with my wife, Glynis, who is an internist. This perspective involves caring for the whole person, to heal the patient's mind, body, and spirit.

Previously considered an alternative therapy, but now mainstream, mind-body treatments are being heralded for preventing and treating disorders from diabetes to cancer. This holistic approach plays a daily role in our respective practices, where we have seen firsthand the benefits from treating the individual not as a body to be mechanically fixed, but as a nuanced being to be artfully healed.

SheaNetics, as a lifestyle, wellness, and excercise practice, fits perfectly within this revolutionary approach, promoting personal health and well-being from the inside out. Having practiced it ourselves, we can confirm the challenging nature of the program and its effectiveness.

Its 5 Living Principles: Commitment, Perseverance, Self-Control, Integrity, and Love, are applicable to all ages and have been specifically crafted to bring about great changes physically, mentally, and emotionally. Working primarily with cancer patients, I immediately recognized the power of this practice within a health-care setting. Its ability to inspire hope can work wonders with those struggling with the physical and emotional ramifications of cancer. SheaNetics can be a vital tool in maintaining a healthy, disease-free lifestyle with sound mental and emotional well-being.

We invite you to experience what we have found to be an incredible advance in our medical awareness of the human body. May SheaNetics grant you great peace of mind, strength of body, and wholeness of spirit.

Pankaj Vashi, M.D.
Chief, Department of Surgery
National Director–Gastroenterology & Nutrition Metabolic Support
Cancer Treatment Centers of America at Midwestern Regional
Medical Center, Zion, Illinois

Glynis Vashi, M.D.
Internist, New Patient Clinic Cancer Treatment Centers of America
at Midwestern Regional Medical Center, Zion, Illinois

Introduction

If you are holding this book in your hands, you are probably looking for some type of change in your life that brings clarity, meaning, and enrichment. Before I share with you how you can achieve valuable transformation by experiencing personal Breakthroughs, I'd like to tell you about my journey.

I am a fitness expert, professional trainer, and wellness coach with a lifetime of mind-body experience and a passion for health and well-being. This passion inspired me to create SheaNetics®, a revolutionary wellness-awakening lifestyle practice that blends Eastern and Western values and movements to unite the mind and body as one. SheaNetics brings you a fresh new approach to excercise with a self-styled combination of yoga, Pilates, tai chi, martial arts, GYROKINESIS®, dance, and more. It features the body-enhancing benefits of Tri-Core Power Training, a highly effective technique for developing all three regions of your core to improve balance and boost physical performance.

In addition to exercising your body, it is critical to engage both mind and heart in the process. For this reason, the grounding philosophy of a SheaNetics lifestyle centers on the practice of The 5 Living Principles of Well-Being as its inspirational answer to living the life you have always wanted: Commitment, Perseverance, Self-Control, Integrity, and Love. These Principles are the keys to creating and maintaining a personal state of well-being. With SheaNetics, you get in shape, feel great about yourself, and naturally come to embrace ongoing life-healthy choices.

Although many of us seek the health and balance that comes through creating harmony within our minds, bodies, and hearts, finding well-being can seem as challenging as climbing Mount Everest. It's really more like Dorothy in *The Wizard of Oz*, who clicked her heels and realized the answers she had been searching for were there all along—just as SheaNetics is there for you.

This book is an extension of my classroom and training, where I share and listen to stories about how The 5 Living Principles of Well-Being have opened doors for so many of my students and friends. I hope that this book will wake up your heart. My wish is to encourage you to look inside yourself and ask, "Am I ready for my Breakthroughs? Am I ready to admit the things I need to do in order to have the health and peace of mind I am looking for? Am I ready to put a plan together and to start living it? Am I ready to Embrace It, Own It, Live It®?"

What is a Breakthrough? Have you ever had a moment or a period in your life when you just seemed to "get it"? That is, at first you saw something in a certain way and were not open to considering alternate views, then all of a sudden for some reason it took on a new importance or your perspective changed, opening a doorway to understanding. It is like flipping a switch. A Breakthrough can happen any day, week, month, or year. The bulb goes on, and with it comes enlightenment.

In this book, I'll explain how Breakthroughs do one of two things: they either confirm that we are on the right track or confirm that we are on the wrong track. It is usually easier to keep our heads down and just keep doing what we've always done—until we have no choice but to look up, and there it is: smack! It's right in our faces, and we have no option but to address what we have tried to avoid. Breakthroughs are a proactive and positive way to take more control of your life; to confront your challenges and pursue your desires and dreams; and to finally reach out for the truth, help, and fulfillment you have been longing to find.

"Embrace It,

Own It,

Live It®"

The process of self-discovery and finding well-being is very personal, and the road traveled is different for each of us. In this book I share my journey, but what I hope will be of greatest benefit to the reader are the powerful tools I have found that work for me and the others who have embraced them. Are you ready? Let's begin.

CHAPTER ONE

What Is a Breakthrough?

"The most exciting breakthroughs
of the twenty-first century will not occur because
of technology but because of an expanding
concept of what it means to be human."

—John Naisbitt

When my students come in to take a class, I like to start by thanking them for making the commitment to show up. In picking up this book and reading these very first words, you have made a commitment. A commitment to yourself. Maybe it comes from your curiosity, interest, or just an inner sense that the way you are living is leaving you unfulfilled and doubtful of the course you are on. In essence, you are on a search that has brought you here. I invite you to experience what I have to share about creating the healthful and balanced lifestyle you seek—your new life of well-being.

As you read, it is important for you to quiet the concerns and stresses that distract or weigh you down. When people enter my studio, I always ask them to leave their challenges, concerns, or stresses at the door because they will be waiting for them when class is over. Have you ever gone to sleep with a sink full of dirty dishes and awakened to a clean and empty one? Wouldn't that be nice? The grit and grime will always be there, but right now, this is your time. Setting aside whatever concerns or worries you might have prepares you to be "in the moment." Being in the "here and now" is not about what you did or didn't do before this time, nor what you might do later on. To have the best experience possible—mentally and physically—you must readjust your focus and concentration to what you are about to do. This act begins a meditative process whereby the redirection of thoughts and actions transforms the activity into a positive and therapeutic experience. You can begin to do this in little ways. Use the act of turning this page as a metaphor for clearing the clutter in your head. Just turn and clear.

To some people who only come expecting a workout it may seem odd to ask them to fully reorient themselves mentally for the class. After all, if they didn't want to be there, they wouldn't have shown up, right? But if you think about it, aren't we all so hurried in our lives and going through the motions that we are barely present in any of the things we do, whether they are tedious errands or projects at work or driving in traffic or something as pleasant as an exercise class? Our sights are set on multitasking. Ever eat breakfast while driving to work? Ever check your child's homework while on hold with the credit card company? Ever sit in a restaurant with a guest who is constantly checking her BlackBerry or texting? Ever have someone talk to you without you hearing a word? *I'm sorry, could you repeat that again? My head was somewhere else.* Ever read the same paragraph in a book twice and still not know what it said? You get the picture.

We are constantly ahead of ourselves, never fully engaged, and ultimately, because of that, we get in our own way. After a while, nothing we do seems to have rhyme or reason. Perhaps that is because our full mental engagement is lacking and we can't appreciate the importance of what we are doing or even what we want to accomplish in the first place. Our minds become like one big giant traffic jam. You can't move in any direction, you don't have any plans for an alternate route, and yet you want to get to your destination as quickly as possible, because if you don't, you are afraid you might miss something.

The big problem that follows this kind of pattern is *what is really NOT worth missing has already passed.* You perform in a robotic perfunctory way without any understanding of the relevant context of life that surrounds your actions or the meaning within them. I think we can agree—while you may be alive, you have missed your opportunity and that is not really "productive living."

As women we are especially susceptible to a life that feels this way. We want to be our best. We try our very hardest from the minute we wake up to the minute we go to bed (if we even sleep!) to lose weight; get in shape; get that promotion; be a better mother, daughter, friend, student, spouse, person. Go higher, do more, and look terrific doing it. I spent years as a wife, mother, and career woman multitasking and oblivious to the value of being in the moment. I was always thinking about the next task, the next business deal, the next event . . . the next, the next . . .

Until I had a Breakthrough.

I realized where you are right now is more important than where you are going. Our true purpose in life is usually more elusive than what we believe it to be. We should continue to plan for tomorrow, but it is not something over which we have exact control. There are so many variables that can potentially come into play. So while we plan for the future, we also need to make the most of today. The focus becomes on how to live in the moment the best way we can, and, frankly, for many of us, this is much easier said than done. What I have found, however, is that each of us possesses the tools to do this. Some of us just need a little more help in finding these tools and putting them to good use.

All we want is for it to all click into place. We want to know the efforts we are making will pay off in the end, despite the fact that our pace may be slowly killing us mentally, physically, and emotionally. We ask ourselves, *When will it all happen? When will my hard work pay off? What will it take to make me happy?* And in the meantime, we give credence to these internal voices that tell us to go farther, faster, or else nothing we do will ever be good enough. The self-criticism never ceases and sweeps us into a stress-filled abyss, and then a phenomenon occurs: We begin to *believe* we aren't good enough, and then we stop. Our fears become self-fulfilling. The harder we push, the more we wish; the longer we try, usually ends with our giving up. We can't sustain the path on which we have set ourselves because it is too rigorous, too unforgiving, and is not rooted in a true understanding of who we are and why we want all of these things in the first place, or if we even truly want them at all. And a vicious cycle is born: we try and then we try harder until we exhaust ourselves and we have to halt. We resolve and then resign. We struggle to follow through. We become discouraged and insecure. At the same time, we may attempt to buoy ourselves through overindulgence in food, liquor, and even drugs, which ultimately works against us.

If this sounds like you, it's time for a Breakthrough of your own. But what exactly is a Breakthrough? It is a change in the way you view something; it can be a subtle or radical shift in perception. It may be a change in how you have thought about someone or something, especially perhaps the perception you have of yourself and of what you are (or are not) capable. It is the moment of realizing a truth, and even small changes can have profound effects. When the lightbulb that has been flickering finally goes on—and stays on—that's when you finally get it.

We are creatures of habit and tend to look at our lives, ourselves, and others in a certain way, through a certain lens. But then one day, you see it differently. For your entire life you were only able to look at something in one way, and then one day life steps in—*whack!*—and you become tuned in to receive a different message about how you view things. A new doorway to understanding is opened, for better or for worse.

In its simplest terms, a Breakthrough is clarity, the kind that leads to true understanding and objectivity. When you see clearly, you can see the sky in its entirety—all the way to the horizon—and lasting change becomes possible. Breakthroughs knock us off the cycle of well-intended beginnings that end quickly with the same unfulfilled results. And that's powerful.

The good news is that Breakthroughs don't have to be these big epiphanies in which your whole life changes instantly. Even the Buddha wasn't enlightened overnight. He had to suffer and be exposed to an ugly world, in which his sheltered princely beliefs about humanity and reality were broken open, changed forever because he finally saw things differently from what he always believed them to be—he saw things for what they *really* were—and experienced enlightenment through this clarity. He had a Breakthrough!

Breakthroughs can be small and seemingly insignificant, like the realization that simply eliminating soda from your diet can help you lose weight and avoid type 2 diabetes. Or it can be huge, like the one I had that I will share with you shortly. How big or small a Breakthrough is doesn't matter. What a Breakthrough must do, though, in order for it to be truly meaningful, is to evoke thought and impart change. It allows you to step back and honestly assess how you feel about yourself, see others, and evaluate the challenges in front of you. It gives you the strength to then move forward and ignite your personal power to live a healthier life.

Shea's Breakthrough

My parents, Jeanette and George; my sister, Gail; my brother, Jerry; and I lived in Brantford, Ontario, Canada, and when I was seven years old, my mother divorced my father. My father was often described as the type of man who could get dropped off naked in the middle of New York City with nothing and still survive and thrive. But his devices fell short when it came to loyalty, love, and family. Let's just say he was not the most devoted and caring father or husband.

My father grew up in true poverty, and he lived his life trying to live that fact down. Dad was in the jewelry business, and one of his diversions, besides women and playing poker or the horses, was to go each year to the Toronto Exhibition Place where he would barter for the collectible Gibson Dolls. In that time, Gibson Dolls were every girl's wish—beautiful handcrafted works of art. He would bring them home and set them up on the couch in the living room and show them off, but we girls were never allowed to even touch them. In our young heads it created such yearning and confusion because we never understood why.

George's world was all about him. He would buy custom-made suits and new Cadillacs. It made him feel good to have all eyes on him, the envy of all who met him. He felt he had "arrived." I can remember one winter afternoon when I was maybe seven years old, my sister and I were walking home from her violin lesson when our father saw us in the street. He passed right by us in his Cadillac and wouldn't pick us up because we were not allowed in the car. However, when we got home we were punished because we got our boots and feet wet from walking in the snow. He started to beat my sister with a belt and I lay across her so she would not get hit. My father said, "If you're stupid enough to take the punishment for her then here it is!"

George got exactly what he wanted in life—money, possessions, toys, validation—and to do it he overlooked the most precious thing in life. We missed out on being Daddy's girls, but he missed out on the special love that only comes with being a family.

When my mother divorced my father she left with only what she could pack in our suitcases. Mom moved Gail and me to Ohio, where I spent the rest of my childhood. My mom was the daughter of my grandfather's first wife, and he still lived in Ohio, but the practical reason we came back to the States was work: Mom was a hairdresser, just like her father, George—yes, another one. When we arrived in the small town of Buckeye Lake, Ohio, we had no place to stay and little money.

Arriving in Buckeye Lake, under lean circumstances, we found there was no room for us at Grandfather's. His house was full. He had remarried for the fifth time to a much younger woman and they had two daughters. So our only option at the time was to settle into living quarters in the back of his beauty shop, and for a good while my sister and I slept on chairs we put together. While we might have been a bit disappointed and felt conditions were maybe a little less than ideal, we found later this was a blessing in disguise, which I will discuss further in Chapter 2. Meanwhile, my brother, Jerry, who was nine years older than me, stayed in Canada. Sadly, as a result of this arrangement we seldom saw him until about five years later when he moved to where we had relocated in Newark, Ohio.

My father never sent Mom any money or child support. The responsibility for taking care of us fell solely on her, so she had no choice but to work all her life and did so until the age of sixty-four. I can remember growing up and thinking how nice it would be to have my mom home making cookies and waiting for me to walk through the door after school. Instead, my sister and I did most of the cleaning and cooking during the week.

Mom was always a hard worker, and shortly after moving to Ohio she ventured out on her own to open two salons and later a beauty school in Newark. Through this period we still lived in a pretty small town, but over time Mom and her businesses were steady. She was able to manage a one-bedroom apartment where we were happy to graduate from our chairs to a place of our own even though the three of us had to share the same bed. Mom saved and later purchased a three-bedroom ranch house where I spent most of my early years.

After my mother divorced my father he lived with Bert, a woman he stayed with for about ten years. My father had always pursued an extracurricular lifestyle, and the fact he had been seeing Bert while he was still married to my mother made their breakup inevitable. Bert and my father set up house. The two of them had three children together: my half sisters and brother, Linda, Marion, and Gary. All during George and Bert's relationship he continued to pursue his regular lifestyle, coming and going as he pleased. He enabled Bert's addiction to alcohol, which contributed to her personal downfall. Eventually, they too split because of Bert's inability to take care of her children. Linda left home, Gary went to live with my father, and Marion, the youngest, wound up in foster care. Bert lost everything.

Interestingly, eleven years after my mother divorced my father, she remarried him. It was just a few years after my first marriage and she honestly believed he was a different person.

When my mother got back with my father, she selflessly took all three of Bert's children in and helped raise them. I can remember asking my mother why. She said, "They are the gifts that came from the relationship; they are just children who need a home and love." And the gift continues giving. Today I enjoy a wonderful relationship with my half sisters and brother, although they all still live in Canada.

My parents' second marriage ended in a separation with my father living in Canada and Mom staying in Florida where they had spent their winters. Mom's explanation for their parting was "Your dad had not changed at all. He just got older and slowed up."

My mother had accumulated Social Security benefits over the years through her work in the States. My father had remained in Canada and had always been self-employed in the jewelry business. By the time Mom retired at age sixty-four she was sharp and alert as ever but physically worn-out. She had osteoporosis. She could not, by any means, have continued to work, and since George never felt it was his obligation to send her any support, she had to rely completely on her Social Security payments. They were not much to begin with, but the situation was aggravated because the law allowed my father, who was still married to Mom but separated for years and living in Canada, to collect half the amount my mother received.

Shortly after Mom retired, she had a conversation with my father about the checks he was receiving. Since he had been working all these years and never paid child support or alimony or support of any kind since their separation, he promised Mom he would do the gentlemanly thing and put her Social Security money that he received in an account for her and then send her a monthly check.

Mom allowed this last lie of his to continue and not seek yet another divorce from him. Perhaps, in part, it was because of the toll on her of so many emotional years with my father, as well as maybe naively thinking he would ultimately keep his word about sending her the money. He never did. In any event, years went by and no funds ever came. So my sister Gail and I decided to go to Canada and confront my father. In our eyes he was not entitled to this money. In our minds, it was morally hers, and he had agreed to give it to her. So we went to confront our father and fight for our mom because her health would not allow her to do it herself.

We met up in Canada with Linda and Marion, my half sisters, and the four of us went to speak with my father. My sister, Gail, came up with the idea to meet with our father first, separately, feeling as the eldest sister she might be able to better persuade him. But she was ambushed. He turned the meeting completely around into a judgment of her. The ongoing problem was he was the master of manipulation. Through the years, no matter what he'd done or failed to do—which was anything at all for us—or how abandoned we might have felt, each of us kids continually sought his approval but never received it. But we weren't there for the past. We had come on an errand of mercy for our mother; to defend the woman who single-handedly raised us and needed our help. Together we all went back inside to meet with him again.

I immediately said to him, "You made a promise to Mom and you never kept it." *Didn't he feel any obligation toward her?*

"Well, she was the one who left me," he said.

"How could anyone stay with you living the life you did?" I asked. "Only thinking of yourself . . . without taking any responsibility for anyone. . . . You fathered three children with Bert and never married her, and Marion ended up in a foster home."

"If it hadn't been for Mom," I continued, "coming back to you after I got married and taking them all in and helping to raise them, who knows where they would be today?"

"I don't intend to pay the money back to your mother," he stated flatly.

"Why?"

"If I didn't deserve to get it, the government wouldn't be giving it to me."

"That's not the point," I retorted. "The point is you promised Mom . . . she never asked *you* for anything *you* had earned . . . and she was the one who'd worked all those years to get the Social Security."

But my father did not play on the field of logic and fundamental fairness. He would change the subject to something more convenient for him.

"Look, you seem to have the need to have a relationship with me. So if you need to have a relationship with me, then that is your decision because I have never needed to have a relationship with you—any of you."

Whack!

A light went on.

I'd never really thought about it in those terms. It was as if I were hearing these words for the first time. His message truly penetrated because I was tuned into what he was saying. I was "in the moment"—my mind wasn't clouded by my own thoughts and judgments. I wasn't feeding myself lies or justifications for his actions. I was clear. I stayed calm. And this clarity allowed me to see the situation for what it really was, and, therefore, prompted a Breakthrough: My father did not have a conscience and would never grow one, so this conversation was over, once and for all. He wasn't capable. And there was nothing I could do about it. It was certainly a big disappointment we would not be able to help our mother. In reality, it was more our journey than hers. She'd already accepted the outcome and might have been surprised had it been any different. My Breakthrough was realizing I would just have to learn to come to grips with the situation and move on knowing my father never loved me or likely any of us.

Most times it is easier to keep our heads down and keep

doing what we always do until we have no choice but to look up, and there it is—*boom*—right in our face. And we have no option but to address what we have tried to avoid. This is not necessarily a bad thing. On the contrary, only good can come from finally confronting your problems, demons, or weaknesses. There is nothing bad in reaching out for the truth. Embarking on such a journey can be healthy, cleansing, energizing, and life affirming, as the Breakthrough I had regarding my father was for me.

The wonderful thing about Breakthroughs is that they provide a priceless gift: freedom. Once you see a person or situation for what it really is, liberation occurs. My Breakthrough with my father offered me freedom. I realized after the hurt, pain, and crying was over that I really did not need him. I only thought all those years that I did. It was hard to get my head around it at first, because as a child, regardless of what your parents have done (or haven't done), you naturally seek their love and validation. Once I knew the truth, I had a Breakthrough, which changed my perception of him and the situation. I consciously and subconsciously could stop putting any thought or effort into hoping and waiting for him to change, to come around, to be the man we could only wish for him to be. Now my time, energy, and mind were *free* for other things. The answers to this problem had been found, and with that, a weight was lifted from my shoulders. My Breakthrough allowed me to release so much bad energy and make space for new and better things to come into my life.

And this is what I hope for you—to experience a radical shift in how you perceive yourself and find freedom from self-limiting thoughts and behaviors, negative self-talk, and unrequited dreams and goals, *and see yourself for who you really are*—committed, strong, vibrant, loving, loyal, gifted, and deserving of the very best life has to offer. This is your Breakthrough, and once you have it, you will be ready to seize the immense greatness that is within you and fully capitalize on your personal power.

Shea Vaughn's Breakthrough is about learning how to live in the moment. When you live in the moment, you are more positive, more motivated, more directed, and free from self-limitations and negative self-talk. When you live in the moment, you set aside your fear and learn to recognize what you can control and what you can't. Now doesn't this sound like the kind of place you want to be so you can make real and life-lasting changes?

This book presents the idea of living in the moment or "mindfulness" as an influence of Eastern thinking and an impetus to experiencing Breakthroughs in our lives. Breakthroughs are shifts by degrees in perception that come from moments of clarity when we are able to put our minds and bodies into healthier, more relaxed, more proactive states. It is a mental and emotional cycle—very different from the Sisyphean effort to change George's mind described earlier in this chapter. We call it the "Anatomy of a Breakthrough": the more focused, clear thinking, and calmer we are, the more presence of mind we achieve; this gives way to greater awareness and the ability to more effectively assess and evaluate our perceptions, leading us to realizations that open the door to experiencing Breakthroughs.

With this positive, new synergistic cycle, anything becomes possible—you can channel away stress, build endearing and enduring relationships, get in shape, feel good about yourself, and naturally embrace a healthy lifestyle.

I believe we are all here to learn certain lessons, and the sooner we can break through our shortcomings, or whatever it is that holds us back, the sooner we can move on to a more fulfilling and loving life.

I hope this book will wake up your mind, body, and heart. My wish is to encourage you to look inside yourself and ask the questions: *Am I ready for my Breakthroughs? Am I ready to admit the things that I need to do in order to find the health, well-being, and peace of mind I am looking for? Am I ready to put a plan together and start to live it? Am I ready to change the way I see myself? Do I want to be free to grow as a person? Am I ready to* **Embrace It, Own It, Live It®**?

If your answers are all yes, then this is your time to turn the page.

"Embrace It,

Own It,

Live It®"

CHAPTER TWO

What's in a Moment?

"With the past, I have nothing to do;
nor with the future.
I live now."

—Ralph Waldo Emerson

Have you ever noticed that in our haste to make the deadline, the journey is often forgotten, and with it, the meaning and enjoyment to be found in each step along the way? We know life is made up of moments, but being aware of that and what happens in each one

enables us to escape—if only for a time—the confusion and emptiness that haste and disorder can create. This awareness also enables
us to connect more deeply with who we *really* are, how we feel, what
we hope to do, or even how we plan to do it. It is important, too, to
understand that "what's in a moment" is a matter of stages, and they
can take you anywhere, from just catching your breath to understanding the profound. Notably, it can be a powerful gateway to finding the
balance, fulfillment, and happiness we all seek. This is what the gift of
life is all about.

Breakthroughs are manifested through an integrated synergistic cycle that begins by creating presence of mind or "living in the
moment." This was introduced briefly in our last chapter as the Anatomy of a Breakthrough.

The Anatomy process begins by being present, but what does this
mean? It is the state or ability to focus, perceive, feel, or to be conscious of an object, sound, sense, event, or anything that helps you
tune out everything else. It sounds so simple, but for many of us,
we find that our consciousness of things and events—both big and
small—that fill our moments is sabotaged by the stressors in our
lives. But there is a way to learn to invite the moment back into your
consciousness, through what I call The 5 Living Principles of Well-
Being, which you will be formally introduced to in Chapter 5; along

with helpful advice in Chapter 6 on how to usefully apply them in your life. But first . . . a bit more about presence and its relationship to Breakthroughs.

Creating Presence

The Anatomy of a Breakthrough begins with "presence of mind," or "being present." These terms are synonymous with the Eastern notion of mindfulness. All cultures value mindfulness, being present, or in the moment, or even "in the zone," as athletes often call it. It has different names but means the same thing. Presence is about being able to tune out the noise around you (stressors) to focus in a different direction. This sets the stage for the next step through, which you can become aware and acknowledge what you are doing, its meaning, and the ability to experience a given time in your life. To do so adds context and richness to your existence.

Presence is about being able to tune out the noise around you.

Being Aware of Awareness

Becoming aware does not mean having everything revealed at once. In fact, it can take many moments over time for this to occur. Nonetheless, most of us can use tools to help us gain awareness and focus on what we are doing at a given time; to slow things down and evaluate where we are and where we are going. That's where The 5 Living Principles of Well-Being come in (which, as I mentioned, we'll explore thoroughly in upcoming chapters).

People think and say they are paying attention; however, they are often really doing just the opposite—running around having the same hectic days, years, and lives. Their schedule is driving them instead of them driving their schedule. There is no time for a moment of awareness or reflection let alone the realization that some changes need to be made.

Being in the moment is a conscious decision and a reminder to yourself that you have to evoke that level of presence and awareness. When you do this often enough, you get to the point where you can tune in to that place inside yourself more easily without the reminders. Most everyone is familiar with the saying, "Stop and smell the roses." It is a friendly admonishment to slow down and appreciate the things around you, or the simple pleasures in life. At its basic level, doing so puts you "in the moment."

In and of itself this pause is meditative, as it gives you a break from stress by diverting your attention to something meaningful. Maybe it's just the act of breathing in and exhaling slowly or a brief acknowledgment of the pleasant reality that you are alive. However, at the next level it opens the door to a contemplative state that invites self-observation and assessment. This is the third phase in the Anatomy and is where you really get the chance to engage in meaningful observation, evaluation, and self-discussion that empowers realization, breakthrough, and change. But unless you have some trigger, how many busy people remember to do it or have the tools necessary to enable them?

In Chapter 4, I will discuss more fully the meditative process and its importance in guiding you toward a life of mindfulness and awareness. In Chapter 5, we will look at The 5 Living Principles of Well-Being as practical tools to use anytime and anywhere. They will help you see the potential and vitality in every moment, build on each one, and connect them in ways that can powerfully enhance your life by guiding your decisions and reshaping your future actions in meaningful ways.

So, if living in the moment or being aware is so vital to Breakthroughs, then what exactly is *in* a moment that makes it so powerful and life changing? Because such an answer is certainly not going to be a single, standard response, I turned to some students and friends and asked them, "What's in a moment?" Here are a few of the answers they shared:

"Every possibility on earth."

"Infinite chances for improvement."

"Nothing and everything."

"My life as I know it."

"As good as it gets."

"*I* am the moment."

"Temporariness."

"Life itself."

"Second, third, fourth chances . . . "

"Miracles."

"Wisdom."

Whatever you feel best describes it, one thing is for certain: moments can be anything. But empirically, every moment, whether it's one of good fortune (or not), brings us truth and hope. Truth is the reality in a moment of who or where we are and how we feel or react to it; and hope is there as an offer or promise of a Breakthrough now or in some future moment.

You may recall in what modest fashion my mom, Gail, and I were introduced to Buckeye Lake when we first came from Canada. That changed briefly for us just before we were able to afford an apartment when Grandfather asked us to come and stay with him. He was married for the fifth time to a much younger woman with whom he'd had two daughters, Georgia Ann and Kathy Jo. In due time, I learned that his ideas and habits were not much different than my father's, except Grandfather had a streak in him that was just plain mean. Georgia Ann and Kathy Jo were within two years in age of my sister and me. So, although they were our aunts, they were more like sisters to us in terms of age.

We soon learned that Grandfather took great pleasure literally pitting his two girls in wrestling matches against my sister and me where "anything went." He looked at them more as the sons he never had and took joy in proving they were tougher and stronger than us. Luckily, as I mentioned above, our stay with our grandfather was short, which actually turned out to be a blessing, and while we still didn't fully escape the "matches" he instigated between us girls, we no doubt dodged much of the unhealthy mental and physical affects his dysfunctional behavior might have otherwise had on us.

The truth is that while our beginnings in Buckeye were not ideal, by mostly living separately from my grandfather and his family we were spared the full brunt of his darker personality. Yes, we had to accept our accommodations in the back of the beauty shop for what they were, but thankfully we had a roof over our heads. We also had hope for the future. With a place to stay and a means for Mom and later my sister and me to make a livelihood, we had a solid chance to improve the condition and quality of our lives. We also learned there is always hope for family, and today my sister and I have a loving relationship with Georgia Ann and Kathy Jo.

Our journeys to lasting change are not easy, but knowing that truth and hope are present in everything we do and exist in every outcome helps us find courage to continue our pursuit. Sometimes the truth is tough to take—about ourselves or others—but when we find the strength to truly face it, we are rewarded with the hope that always follows. Where there is truth there is hope; hope that whatever we need to acknowledge will get better, and that we can be the power behind making a change. When you allow truth and hope to lead you, you will find you are less afraid of looking at things with your eyes wide open (truth) and can begin to look for brighter days ahead (hope).

Truth and hope are in each moment and being aware of their presence helps us to objectively evaluate what we see without fear getting in the way, so we can create the right conditions for Breakthroughs. It comes back to the cycle: the more present we are, the more effectively (truthfully) we can assess and evaluate our perceptions, and the more likely and more often we will be able (hope) to experience Breakthroughs.

To me, what's in a moment is the opportunity for the mind and heart to move forward with awareness, clarity, and caring that bring answers.

Moments can be personal or shared and they do not necessarily have to be positive, hopeful, and good all of the time. In fact, moments that bring on suffering or cause us to react negatively are vital to experiencing Breakthroughs. It's not the essence of the moment; it's the awareness and understanding of it that elicits Breakthroughs. Said differently: it's not what *happens* in the moment, it's what you *notice* is happening that counts.

It makes logical sense to want to live in the moment when that moment is good (*Oh, I wish this moment could last forever.*), but why would we want to be aware of a moment that causes us to react negatively? Why, in effect, would we want to feel ourselves suffering in the moment? What can that contribute to our lives? Loss and grief are inevitable parts of the darkness of suffering, but these are instrumental

It's not the essence of the moment; it's the awareness and understanding of it that elicits Breakthroughs.

33

in experiencing Breakthroughs. When we acknowledge the reality that lightness exists within darkness and vice versa, we see the inter-connectivity of everything—and in that realization comes an under-standing and acceptance of the complex dichotomy of dark and light, of good and evil, of fortune and misfortune. When we approach this interrelationship of things more intellectually, it reduces anxiety and promotes clarity and insight into our situation from which we can make informed choices and more fully anticipate the consequences of our decisions and actions.

Part of the Breakthrough is the further realization that everything we do, good or bad, has a ripple effect on our loved ones, friends, and others; and it is only once we really grasp these effects can we begin to meaningfully help ourselves make better decisions. That is Truth, and once we acknowledge that, we find Hope to build a formula that actually helps us, and will, therefore, help others.

Shea's Breakthrough

Here is a not-so-magic moment that at first caused me great pain, but through awareness of the moment, as bad as it was at the time, I found the Truth and Hope that ultimately led to another valuable Breakthrough in my life.

Growing up as I did, I was fortunate enough to have a mother who was ahead of her time in terms of independence, grace, intellect, and strength. What she wanted for us was to go through beauty school and get licensed so we would have a career to fall back on—something that would sustain us and give us independence. However, my first love in life was always dance and ballet, and I trained and progressed from student to teacher. I also had a dream of going to New York and dancing on Broadway, so marriage was not in my immediate plan. And then . . .

I met Vernon Vaughn and fell madly in love. At six feet two inches tall, he was the most handsome man I had ever seen—a knight in shining armor. He was from nearby Zanesville. We met at a dance held at Buckeye Lake near my home in Newark, Ohio. I went with my older sister, Gail, and her friend, both of whom were already in college. I was a senior in high school and thought it was pretty cool to be hanging out with a college crowd.

When we got to the dance, we found a table and occasionally danced with some boys we already knew. Gail and her friend couldn't stop talking about the two guys sitting a few tables away and how "drop-dead gorgeous they were." Gail was just *dying* to have Vernon ask her to dance.

A few songs later, Vernon and his friend were walking in our direction.

"He's coming over to ask me to dance," Gail whispered, elbowing me feverishly.

But Vernon surprised us both when I felt a tap on my shoulder and turned to face him as he asked me to dance instead. I don't really remember much else since I was so caught up in being the focus of this handsome man's attention. Vernon and I danced several dances together and then on and off for the rest of the evening. He and his friend joined us three girls at the table, and while Gail and her friend danced the night away with various other young men, I spent the rest of the evening dancing and talking with Vernon.

It was love at first sight, and it soon became an exclusive relationship. Vernon was already a senior in college when we met. We were married three years later and had three children, Victoria, Valeri, and Vincent.

We were both pretty young and came from divorced families, so we felt strongly about raising our children without the fallout of that kind of unsettling experience. However, neither one of us had really lived much of life nor were we probably much different from many other young couples who bring childhood baggage along to an intimate relationship. Over time, unfortunately, the buildup of our unresolved issues was enough to upset the apple cart, and our shared dreams crumbled beneath the family we had created. Twenty-three years of marriage ended in divorce.

To see your family break up is a pain that pierces so deeply you feel your heart is broken beyond repair. And on top of that, the love I had for my husband was a wound without repair. Aware and conscious of the repercussions, my Breakthrough began when I realized you can love someone but not necessarily live with him. Tina Turner got it right when she sang, "What's love got to do with it?" Marriage takes more than love. It takes both partners working together with mutual respect and for common goals. It takes loving enough to want to change and giving more than you ever thought possible.

But sometimes this level of maturity is just beyond some of us, and even life and events can simply conspire uncontrollably to defeat your best efforts.

Coming to grips with my need to move on was a challenging and necessary Breakthrough, but what I also had to reconcile were the emotional ripple effects that came along with it. For me there were still lessons to be learned and there would be no peace until I was able to find a way to forgive myself, my spouse, and both of us for all the other hurtful family consequences that occurred during our marriage and accompanied its ending.

At first, still wrapped up in the emotion of the experience, I think most divorced couples just think it is the other spouse's fault. In reality it is not often likely that only one spouse is 100 percent wrong. Looking at yourself and being honest about what part you played to cause the breakup is essential if history is not going to repeat itself. Perhaps if we both had been able to find more patience and better communication skills, if we had early on sought an objective third party for advice . . . "If only" is something we can repeat to ourselves over and over, but that kind of regret is not healthy. We must learn to forgive in order to move forward.

Regardless of the reason, for many of us forgiveness in any form can be one of the toughest things to do. But the Breakthrough is in understanding and coming to peace knowing there are times when some things are just beyond our capabilities. This does not mean making excuses for ourselves. Instead, it is reconciling with the reality and honest truths that we are not perfect. We make mistakes but we need to learn from them, forgive ourselves and others, find a way to live with our decisions, and move forward. None of this is easy.

Once we come to know the truth, there is hope . . . to support our journey forward. Sometimes it is painful and takes much longer than expected or you want it to. But there is more life ahead and you need to live it. That is the Breakthrough.

In moving beyond the resentment and regrets that accompany tragic events like divorce, I was able to assess the situation better and focus my attention on creating the best environment for my children. This led me to my next Breakthrough: realizing that none of this really had to be all about Vernon and me. Over time we were all able to find a way to spend Christmas and other family events together and it didn't matter who had been right or wrong.

You Within the Moment

I have spoken much about awareness of moments, but what about awareness of *you?* Looking at yourself with honesty is essential to ensure history does not repeat itself. As I experienced the above Breakthrough, I found the courage to admit the part I played in the demise of my relationship, decided changes needed to be made that only I could make, and accepted the reality that there are always regrets and hurt in life—an undeniable and unfortunate fact of living life. Once I faced the truth, with new hope I no longer feared the new path I would forge for myself. I found freedom once again; the freedom in knowing you can take moments, positive or negative, and use them to make the next moment even better.

When you are aware of moments, an amazing thing happens: you become aware of yourself. But not the self you think you know; the one who has a meeting or a phone call to return or a few miles to run . . . not the self who picks her kids up at 3:00 PM and then takes them to soccer, and not the self who pays the bills for her elderly parents. The self I am talking about is the one who lives beyond her immediate preoccupations, the one who has been abandoned amidst chaos and stress. How can anyone have a Breakthrough if she doesn't know what her real self wants and needs? All you might know is that you are not happy, you are not living authentically, something is missing. But you can't quite put your finger on it. You are not living with clarity and calmness; only in confusion. Clarity begins with the question, *Who am I?* Do you see who that person is? And if you don't, how can you begin to?

First you need to look past your physicality, beyond what you do for a living, how you've labeled yourself or have been labeled, who you take care of, or what other hobbies or interests you might pursue. This helps you get in better sync with the person you are beyond all the business, the stress, the expectations; the person who possesses the Commitment, the Perseverance, the Self-Control, the Integrity, and the Love to *see* what you are really capable of achieving and then acting on it.

A Breakthrough includes the ability to turn the idea of living in the moment and the awareness that comes from it onto yourself. That means being able to look in the mirror with honesty and say beyond your reflection: I know now who I really am and what I truly want. I have been fortunate enough in my life to have had a Breakthrough that enabled me to stop living in a manner I knew did not reflect who I really was inside. The Anatomy of a Breakthrough, with its guiding Principles, gave me clarity, as it can for you.

Shea's Breakthrough

My mother was a hairdresser and got her cosmetologist license when she was thirteen years old. She loved the industry and it afforded her the opportunity to raise her kids without help from anyone. It gave her independence and she felt it would do the same for her daughters. She also owned and operated her own beauty school. It was a natural progression then for my sister and me to go through my mother's school and for us both to get our cosmetology licenses. In addition, we both worked in one of the beauty shops and taught in the school. However, I couldn't wait until the day was over to go and take a dance class. That is what made me feel alive. I also realized soon after I had received my cosmetology license that this was not the field of choice for me even though it paid the bills.

I discovered that dancing was my love; but as I progressed from student to teacher I also realized that dance teachers taught for the love of it and not for the money. My goal became to find something for which I had a passion that could also provide financial security. I had lived most of my young life in Newark, Ohio, where my mother's beauty school was. By now I had married Vernon, and when he found a job in another town in Ohio, we moved. I missed my family and friends but was excited about building a new life with Vernon and a family of my own.

These changes made me realize I had career choices and how important it was to my personal well-being to find the right fit for me. This was a Breakthrough that helped me throughout the rest of my life. It encouraged me to follow my passion and to be proud about what makes me tick and be able to wake up with the right attitude about living life. I loved being a new mom but also continued with dance and obtained physical fitness accreditations. My husband's job took us to other towns, but through the transfers I would always seek out a local fitness center where, time permitting, I could teach. At first it was dance, and later as each new fitness program evolved, I would get certified as an instructor. While I was perhaps not living an earlier dream of mine to dance on Broadway, I was certainly absorbing a wealth of great choreography and enjoying the journey that would one day provide the building blocks for another big Breakthrough.

The move away from Newark was eye-opening. I was settling into the role of wife and then eleven months later as a new mother, for which I felt blessed. However, I had also learned the value of building something just for yourself that creates self-confidence and balance—something that is unselfishly your own and gives you a sense of accomplishment and fulfillment.

There are times when change is forced upon us, but most often it is an organic process. However, it does not always occur for the right reasons nor may all the ripple effects be immediately visible. For instance, many years later I decided to pursue a career in real estate. The hours were flexible, allowing me to work and still be there for my husband and children. I also really enjoyed meeting and working with my colleagues and clients. The whole process was different, too, from anything I had previously done and I learned a lot about sales and business in general. I also found I had a real empathy for people and a need to help them through what was for many of them the single biggest emotional and financial investment they would ever make.

I was good at the job and successful, but money was never my motivation. What I came to consciously admit much later whether real or imagined, I was seeking Vernon's approval. I allowed this to cloud my thinking and went into the real estate business for all the wrong reasons.

I felt that my worth as a person would be greater to him

because of my accomplishments in that profession. It was not that I was unfulfilled being a wife and mother. I loved my family and worked hard to give them my all. In fact, I wanted to be a stay-at-home mom. But I came to realize that any contribution of mine was not considered by my husband to be of equal value to his contribution as the main breadwinner. It was a perception of his that ran broad-brush and seemed to define our relationship. While there were other issues that frankly were not of his doing, this overshadowed everything, adding to an unfortunate situation that in the end was only able to be resolved by divorce. But along the way, my first Breakthrough was realizing that self-worth and fulfillment are things that come from how you feel about yourself and not by how you are judged by others.

Interestingly, I have continued for years to renew my cosmetology license. It's like having a part of my mom with me, although she is no longer here. It is still not a profession I have ever pursued, but my grandchildren and present husband are now able to reap the benefits. You can't beat haircuts at home! It's a win-win. Their stylist comes to them, and it's a little gift I love giving.

The Power of Awareness

Each of my Breakthroughs began when I allowed myself to be in the moment, to become aware, and to allow myself to experience it—as bad as the moment could be at times. In slowing down and pausing to think it through, I found clarity in each situation, which helped me to examine it for what it really was. My family was breaking up. But there was a new beginning yet to be built—based on a common goal to support our children.

Had I not practiced awareness, I might have stayed resentful, stuck in anger and feeling I was in a hopeless place. Was I completely fulfilled in my career choice? No. But through further self-evaluation I came to a closer understanding of who I am, what inspires me, and what I hoped my life work could be. I certainly felt I had business knowledge and people and communication skills I might not have otherwise had the opportunity to develop, and I would find them valuable in future endeavors. However, in those moments of awareness—of stopping the commotion of external reactions and emotions—I turned inward for a more intellectual version of events. I was able to see things through a truer lens. Stepping out of the emotional responses I had to my divorce or work, I found a center that helped me assess my actions, the actions of others, and how to forge a new path for myself—a Breakthrough, in and of itself, of great meaning to me.

When you are not able to see yourself in life's moments—for who you are, how you feel, what is important to you, or what the moment holds for you—life just kind of drags you along. It becomes more likely for things to just happen to you, and some of these things will be unanticipated, unsettling, and even possibly destructive. When this occurs it can be easy to become anxious, depressed, and addicted to things like food, alcohol, drugs, and sleep aids. This is also how negative cycles can begin. Self-respect disappears and is replaced with self-loathing. Anger and resentment can take over. Sadness prevails. Your body breaks down. Perhaps it's because you can't sleep or eat, or you eat and sleep too much. Disease ensues: high blood pressure, heart disease, obesity, diabetes, phobias—you name it. What's in a moment—our awareness of it and of ourselves in it—is of major importance as it is directly related to our health—mental, physical, and emotional.

Conversely, the clarity that comes with living in the moment nips the negative cycle above in the bud. Overall, physical health is not compromised as easily when you create a state of calmness, focus, and control over your reactions to what life throws at you. In fact, studies have shown that those who achieve mindful living through the practice of meditation ease chronic pain, anxiety, and stress; improve heart health; boost mood and immunity; and resolve pregnancy problems.

How can this be? Why would awareness of the moment and presence of mind create such a healthy physical response, and further, what does that have to do with Breakthroughs? The philosopher Hazrat Inayat Khan said, "Every passion, every emotion, has its effect upon the mind. Every change of mind, however slight, has its effect upon the body." We must be sensitive to the mutual dependency between the mind and body and how our wellness is created through their close affinity and symbiotic relationship. It is in the cultivation of this connection through The 5 Living Principles that we invite life-changing and lasting Breakthroughs into our lives. Let's see how.

CHAPTER THREE

Thought and Motion

A Look into the Mind-Body Connection

*"The fact that the mind rules the body is,
in spite of its neglect by biology and medicine,
the most fundamental fact which we
know about the process of life."*

—Franz Alexander, M.D.

Every day we think. Every day we move. *What* we think and *how* we move very much define who we are. Most of us are constantly barraging ourselves with internal chatter while simultaneously allowing external feedback to infiltrate our minds. Thoughts about ourselves, our dreams, and our ideals are incredibly powerful. They can affect our moods and influence our next thoughts, like dominoes falling in the direction we've stacked them. But our thoughts don't stop there. They also direct our movement. If you see a woman who is walking with her head down, slowly shuffling her feet with her arms crossed across her abdomen, what is your immediate impression of her? Your instinct might be concern or sympathy because her body language seems to call out suffering, sadness, or even defeat.

Thoughts and movement. The two go hand in hand, and each looks to the other for cues on what to do or think next. For instance, have you ever noticed how your body responds to a good report from the boss? What a sweet surge of energy! You move faster, maybe your heart even skips a beat. *Thoughts and movement.*

Have you ever come down with the flu and felt depressed and unproductive because of it? With a bad enough head cold, you can actually convince yourself you may never be able to form a coherent sentence ever again. *Movement and thought.*

I knew a runner once who hurt her knee so badly that she was directed by her doctor to stop running. After quitting the sport, she admitted she felt as if her focus, tenacity, and creativity were dwindling. She thought because she could no longer move in her favorite way, in the way she felt most alive, what she could produce intellectually and emotionally were no longer of value. Sadly, such negative thoughts have a way of becoming self-fulfilling. "All that we are is the result of what we have thought," Buddha once observed. And while Henry Ford put it a little less eloquently, he got to the same point when he said: "Whether you think you can or you can't, you are right."

Our minds and bodies are intricately and inseparably connected, as many great teachers, philosophers, scientists, and authors have told us for centuries, if not since the beginning of time. They have also noted that just because the mind and body are connected, doesn't necessarily mean they are always synergized or synchronized, and therefore we need to nurture the intricate nature of the "mind-body connection" to live a fulfilling, healthy, and happy life.

What Exactly Is the Mind-Body Connection?

The mind-body connection is the idea that our thoughts can positively affect our bodies and our physical reactions, particularly to stress. The mind leads and the body follows. However, there are times the opposite is true. I am so used to vigorous exercise, that after a few days on vacation, while my mind may say, "Let's lay by the pool and read a good mystery," my body's muscles are talking to me saying, "Take me out for a run or let's do some SheaNetics." It's a two-way connection.

If you think back to a time or a place in which you were calm or happy, you will notice your body will respond with a similar good reminiscent feeling. Have you ever walked into a store or some other place where the soothing aroma of incense filled your nose and your senses, and because of a past pleasing association your mind was calmed in that instant? These are examples of the mind-body connection. And while this pleasant scenario can also work in reverse, it is said that making positive connections is a critically important component of attaining and maintaining ultimate well-being.

The brain and the body are connected entities, and should not be cared for as if they operate independently.

The brain and the body are connected entities, and should not be cared for as if they operate independently of one another. Research shows a correlation between many physical and emotional health problems, such as depression and diabetes or post-traumatic stress disorder (PTSD) and cardiovascular disease. In proper form our minds and bodies perform as one.

Practical experience and even neurological research on the topic show this to be the case. Some like to say there are times our minds and bodies "disconnect," and we have to learn how to "reestablish" that lost connection. However, my views differ slightly. As the research suggests there is always a connection, but it may need some "redirection" instead to get you on the right pathway, particularly if you are ever to experience any Breakthroughs.

As we have discussed, presence and awareness are integral factors in achieving Breakthroughs. If our minds and bodies are distracted and engaged in friction, we must find a way to refocus our minds that will help lead our bodies to where we would like to take them: to health, vitality, endurance, and strength. And once we achieve these healthy physical states, our minds are positively affected and create constructive memories that can be "habit forming" in a good way. We like ourselves more, we look for things we know are better for us, we have increased energy, believe more in our abilities, sleep better, and we find freedom from those internal thoughts that keep us bound up in negativity and chaos. It is in this kind of environment we are able to find clarity and calmness—the early conditions of the Anatomy of a Breakthrough, from which Breakthroughs are most possible.

Why Is the Mind-Body Connection Important Anyway? An Introduction to Eastern Philosophy

We live in a Western culture and some say it's *wild* and chaotic here. The individual has usually been conditioned to approach daily life in a compartmentalized way. Each activity is seen as separate from the other, whether it is eating, sleeping, exercising, going to work, or spending time with friends or family, like items to check off a to-do list. But each of these is one of your moments, and they are all connected in a circle of what is your life. Knowing what is happening in each brings context and richness to who you are and the meaning of your existence.

Eastern practitioners have understood the concept of the mind-body connection for eons. The wisdom in their philosophies and teachings has thankfully begun to find a home in some of our Western culture, as evidenced by the increase in interest in mind-body exercise, Ayurvedic medicine, and meditation.

Much of *Shea Vaughn's Breakthrough* has been inspired by Eastern thinking on the subjects of mindfulness, the mind-body connection, and meditation because I have personally experienced and been influenced by the benefits of these teachings and their roles in eliciting

Breakthroughs. Eastern practices help you become aware of the most basic of human actions and their significance. For instance, you would never think of whether or not to breathe or eat. These necessities are automatic; they are simply part of what we do every day. The interesting thing about respiration is that it seems so simple, so natural, so effortless, yet the irony is that awareness of our breathing is one of the most effective tools we have to keep our mind-body connection healthy. This observation is yet one more piece of wisdom given to us from the sages of the East. It is something we will explore more later in this book, and then again when we learn about The 5 Living Principles of Well-Being in Chapter 5.

As I delved a bit deeper into Eastern history, I began to appreciate the guiding precepts of ancient thinking that reflected the reality of those times. There was a class structure and society was governed by a controlling few at the top of the hierarchy. There were no republics, no Congress, no democracy. Patterns of acceptable behavior were dictated partly by absolute decree that was handed down, for which there was no appeal, or by the moral teachings of "wise" or learned thinkers, which evolved more by way of accident than intention. Nonetheless, such teachings imparted a code of living that helped to keep order and provide direction to the collective society.

Most ancient societies also had a martial-warrior class with members guided by a practice that espoused physical discipline and the attainment of mental and moral excellence. It was both a way of life and a circle of life that measured accomplishment and well-being in terms of establishing competence in each of these areas.

This concept is no less practical or relevant today than it was then. I believe it is important for most people to incorporate some kind of philosophy into their lives. It gives direction, purpose, and meaning to what they do and what they experience, and fulfills a basic need we all have for some kind of reassuring structure. We all need something to help remind us, even if it is only occasionally, that following certain teachings, beliefs, and/or moral codes (call it what you will) helps us to be mindful of our actions, to truly live the moments of our lives, enhances each experience, and makes us better people.

Shea's Breakthrough

While I was aware of the mind-body connection, I really didn't understand it on a deep level or incorporate it into my daily life until I enrolled in a martial arts class of Korean origin called Tae Kwon Do. Sometimes the best things in life begin by chance. At the time, my to-be husband, Steve, and stepson, Danny, were already involved in the art. Danny has cystic fibrosis, a hereditary and degenerative genetic disease in children and young adults that affects the entire body, in particular, the lungs, causing progressive disability and often early death. Danny was referred by his doctors to a clinically endorsed martial arts program taught by a black belt in Tae Kwon Do. He had introduced special breathing techniques in an effort to explore the possible therapeutic effects on cystic fibrosis patients. I joined the group later following the conclusion of the study and the three of us continued on at a regular school.

The physical side of class typically included warm-ups, various hand and foot drills, sparring, self-defense techniques, and patterns. The patterns or "poomse" as they are called in Korean are a series of distinctively different choreographed routines of increasing difficulty, which reflect the history of the art as well as the gradual growth of the practitioner's skill. Mastery of each "poomse" would be demonstrated at successive promotion tests and lead to increasing levels of rank and personal responsibility. I approached martial arts as just dancing with force. I thought I "got it" and I would work to bring power to my punching and kicking, refine my balance, and learn some self-defense.

However, at all levels each student was expected to memorize Tae Kwon Do's Seven Tenets—Courtesy, Integrity, Perseverance, Self-Control, Indomitable Spirit, Community Service, and Love—and absorb the history of Korea and the teachings of the founding masters of the art. In the beginning I can remember thinking why and what does memorization have to do with Tae Kwon Do? The physical segment of class was incredibly intense and was followed with us students being directed to sit in a circle. Each in turn was invited by the instructor to share. "What did you get out of the training tonight?" Everyone had a chance to talk and express their thoughts. I remember being a bit surprised the first time someone digressed from the physical to share an experience directly tied to how the Tenets had worked positively in his life.

While the physicality of the experience was certainly a rewarding challenge, the reality of what I expected and what I was experiencing began to change. I found my paradigm shifting from "taking class" to "being a student of the art." I wholeheartedly began to embrace and live the Seven Tenets. I found myself sitting in the circle at the end of each class sharing thoughts about my own personal growth beyond the physical workout I had just completed. What I soon realized was that each class sought to improve the body *and* mind in equal measure—working together to be self-aware and present at all times and pursuing every aspect of life according to a guiding code of conduct.

I finally had a Breakthrough and made the connection that Eastern philosophy promotes adherence to a practice. It was not all about who was the best at doing the patterns, or who I could kick or punch really hard, but how you create balance and enrich the quality of your life and the lives of others. The class did not end after the last punch was thrown. The circle and the verbalizing of what was going on internally and in our minds comprised as much of the class as did the physical exertion—a living example of the mind-body connection being nurtured, executed, and further encouraged to be an integral part of everything we do.

The Mind-Body Conundrum in the Western World

Women in particular have always been concerned about matters physical, emotional, and of what we call the heart. We are hardwired that way, and what tends to happen to any one of us who is also challenged to multitask is that issues remain unresolved, fester, and usually begin to boil over before they get the proper attention. My hope is to help women to change all of that, so we recognize our issues and realize that now is the time to take action.

If you are overweight a little or a lot, fatigued and listless, restless in spirit, have high blood pressure, are borderline or already diabetic, have suffered a heart attack or the doctor has told you you're at risk of having one—if you've experienced any of these and more—then your body is clearly putting your mind on notice that you need to face making some adjustments in your life—at the very least in your diet and your approach to exercise. If you are unhappy at work or at home, have troubled relationships with family, friends or others, bear regrets or disappointments, then they will conspire to deprive you of a healthy mind-body connection and any real possibility of finding well-being.

Emotionally, all of these illnesses and issues can cause stress, the number one cause of so many diseases. It is like a domino effect; your mind and its emotions play a part in your overall physical appearance and negative thinking leads to inaction. "I am too upset to work out." "I can't concentrate on anything else until I resolve this issue." So now you are convinced you cannot do anything positive to help yourself until you take care of this issue—and of course the next and the next.

These are excuses that are just so easy to make and so devastating to our personal well-being. Many times we even know the truth of what we are doing to ourselves and feel guilty about it, but we lack the tools to break the cycle. We do not allow ourselves (or give ourselves permission) to move forward. Knowledge and understanding is key to turning it all around. Our hearts are waiting for our minds to catch up and take control of our emotional and physical disconnect so that our hearts can beat with love and not with speed.

The mind-body connection begins when someone mentally decides to change something, create something, accomplish something, or do something that he or she is not currently doing or has not accomplished thus far. Many people have a want or need to make differences in their lives, in their appearances, and to have a more fulfilling relationship with others, but they just procrastinate or don't know how to do it. However, when the mind takes control the body will follow. That is a mind-body connection. But you must embrace the reality that the responsibility to make it happen is yours alone. When you are mentally willing to initiate a plan and seek help in order to successfully accomplish the goal, the body will follow along working in tandem for your benefit.

A positive mind-body connection has been shown to:

- Decrease anxiety
- Facilitate sleep
- Lessen pain
- Decrease the necessity for medications
- Build the immune system and foster faster healing
- Increase self-confidence and emotional well-being

But creating the connection is not necessarily the only end point. The Anatomy of a Breakthrough describes a sequence of conscious dots to follow: attaining presence of mind, becoming aware, and conducting assessment and evaluation, which lead to realization and the goal of Breakthrough. Any Breakthrough is valuable but not every one produces change, and that is how we enhance our lives—by making mind-body connections that cause us to take action and thereby reap the benefits of our effort. This is the essential goal of pursuing "Your Pathway to Well-Being," and helping you to accomplish this through a synergy of thought and motion is the cornerstone of my Breakthrough methodology SheaNetics.

I was getting ready to teach a small 6:00 AM class one early morning, when Allison walked in and asked, "Am I in the right place?" I answered, "Yes, if you are here to take SheaNetics." Allison had heard about the class and wanted to check it out but was not familiar with its range of purpose as a lifestyle practice.

As class began she listened closely as I explained to everyone The 5 Living Principles of Well-Being (Commitment, Perseverance, Self-Control, Integrity, and Love). Shortly thereafter, we all settled in and I began to teach the class. When it was over Allison came up to me and expressed how much she had enjoyed it and that she was planning to come back on a regular basis.

She kept her Commitment and came to class regularly, which gave us an opportunity to chat together after class. I learned Allison was going through some major changes and challenges in her life: a divorce, a job change, a daughter with whom she had always been close who now didn't want to talk to her, along with diets she started and stopped, and an overall feeling that everything in her life was falling apart.

Allison told me she had tried several diets, each time taking some diet pill that promised, "This is the one"... that will help you lose those extra pounds without having to change any other habits in your life.

Just pop the pill. Nothing worked, and discouraged, she even put on more weight. Allison also shared she was going to counseling to help her deal with the divorce and her estrangement from her daughter. I felt the pain of her challenges.

Several months passed and Allison was now taking my class about twice a week. I noticed that physically she looked more toned. A few days later I ran into her at the local grocery store and we started to talk. As I complimented her on her progress, she told me how she feared the improvements she was making would not last. I shared with her that in order to experience a Breakthrough she needed to engage her mind in her pursuit of a healthier lifestyle. I explained that her body was going through the motions, but she had to get her mind to buy into her plan. I said, "Your mind needs to make the commitment that something needs to change." Why? "Because when the mind leads, the body will follow."

Recapturing what you have lost or gaining what you hope to achieve, takes life-altering changes. The driving force behind it all is your mind and will. It takes hard work and it doesn't happen overnight. We have heard this before but sometimes when we hear it again with a more determined mind-set, it takes on a whole new meaning. Commit to do the work, not by taking some pill but by making a lifestyle change, and you will begin to see the results.

Allison did just that, and as the year progressed I was witness to her Breakthrough. She changed her habits and enjoyed eating healthy food, adding more fruits and vegetables to her diet. She was exercising at least three to four times a week. She found the patience to stop pushing her daughter to do it her way and instead just let her daughter know she loved her and was there for her. She persevered through the divorce proceedings and began to move on. Life was coming back together again and she was feeling pretty good about herself.

Thought and movement are interconnected, and a Breakthrough is what elicits action and change.

I had a chance to experience Allison's Breakthrough from the front row and was witness to the hard work one needs to exert in order to see the effects of their efforts grow. The heart sings when the mind and body connect through a common purpose. Your spirits are raised when the mind and body work as one. I also received a gift from this transformation. My invitation to Breakthrough was the reconfirmation that life is what we make it and our minds are the power behind it. "You are not what you eat—you are what you think."

Thought and movement are interconnected, and a Breakthrough

is what elicits action and change. As the mind gains awareness it can assess and evaluate. This leads to the recognition from which a Breakthrough can emerge. This is the final phase in the Anatomy of a Breakthrough. It's the mental process leading the body toward the change you are seeking. The conundrum is we know our well-being is at risk, yet we are still guilty of so much inaction that we seem to willingly sabotage or inhibit our abilities to take full advantage of the mind-body connection.

If we try to understand why we are so prone to inaction, even when we have the best intentions, we can develop a strategy to recognize it before inaction undermines us. The success of our plan rests on finding the tools that enable us to develop a code for living that will fill our lives with Breakthroughs. This kind of empowerment is to be found in The 5 Living Principles of Well-Being I have centered at the heart of my SheaNetics program. You have seen them in action through the stories you have already read in this book. We are close now to learning these Principles and reaping for ourselves their life-enhancing benefits. However, we must first rally our efforts to disengage and derail a persistently ubiquitous condition that seeks continually to inhibit our ability to experience the Breakthroughs we all innately desire and deserve.

CHAPTER FOUR

Modern Meditation

A Strategy Against Stressors

"By overexerting ourselves to grab the brass ring,
we wind up with rust on our fingers."

—*Shea Vaughn*

Wouldn't it be wonderful if we could just shoo stress away, like we would a fly? Shoo, boss. Shoo, bills. Shoo, chores. Shoo, deadline. Our reality though is different. It's not like shooing or killing the fly; our stress won't go away. We face it from the time we shake off the morning cobwebs until our heads hit the pillow at night. It is just a fact of life.

Stress also comes in varying degrees, from minor annoyances to the most debilitating. Nonetheless, we all need some kind of consistent approach or methodology to process these events and prevent them from escalating and taking over.

Stress can also sabotage our ability to experience Breakthroughs because it weakens the mind-body connection, which we explored in the last chapter, so it's important to focus on controlling our reaction to it. When we are overburdened by chronic stress the mind is doing so much work—thinking, worrying, lamenting, overexerting itself with regrets and "what-ifs"—that the body is sometimes left out. You are so stressed, anxious, and/or depressed that shifts in mood may make it hard to get out of bed; you lose your appetite or overeat as a way to comfort yourself; or maybe you forget to take your vitamins, don't feel like going to the gym, or simply lose interest in something you once loved to do. The state of our minds when under chronic stress can lead us to actually neglect our bodies. Now, *that* doesn't make for a very healthy mind-body connection.

When we are overburdened by chronic stress the mind is doing so much work that the body is sometimes left out.

Stress:
What's Bugging You?

Sometimes even the act of managing stress can cause more stress. At times when I have felt anxious and overwhelmed, the more I thought about how I was feeling and what was on my plate, the more stressed I became. When too much is bothering you, you can find yourself either in attack mode or in automatic shutdown. How we react to stress correlates with how much more stress we make for ourselves.

For instance, I'm a firm believer in the saying "haste makes waste," and those who have tried to operate in a mode of anxiety might agree that trying to get things done when under a tremendous amount of stress or pressure can cause a fumble, which only causes more stress. This is because we tend to try to do things quickly, without concentration or focus, solely in reactive mode. I liken this type of stress reaction to reaching for a slippery bar of soap while in the shower. I'm sure you are familiar with the scenario.

You are late for a conference call and the dog needs to be walked and that comment your coworker made yesterday is still bothering you. You go to grab the soap, as you wait for the conditioner to set, and thump! It falls to the floor. Rolling your eyes and huffing and puffing, you drop to your knees and pick up the soap, as it glides and again slips and slides from your right hand to your left and then fumbles back to your right. And then, thump! Again, it falls to the floor. When did holding a bar of soap require the dexterity of a Ringling Brothers tightrope walker? *Slow down*, you say to yourself. Your brain then tells your body, *pick up and hold the soap.* And that's when you do.

You can't manage stress, but you can learn to give it a break. You can assess your stress more clearly and react more effectively—even if it is to simply finish your shower without breaking a leg or preventing the dog from having an accident on the kitchen floor.

Every form of stress can benefit from taking some sort of action to get relief. If you have a chronic condition that causes you to feel unable to participate in even the simplest of daily tasks, I urge you to seek professional help. However, what we want to do is provide the means to handle everything else before it snowballs into something more severe. The intent of this chapter is to deepen your understanding of stress and how reacting negatively to it can impede the Anatomy of a Breakthrough. I hope to help you help yourself take the right steps in countering stress, so you can bring balance and well-being into your life.

A Funny Little Thing About Stress

Biologically, stress is supposed to function as a useful tool. It's a response all humans are programmed with to help us recognize danger and respond to it in ways that can save our lives. Understanding stress can help us make sense of it and turn it on its head. Once we accomplish that, we no longer fear stress; we can learn to use it.

Stress comes from our body's response to danger stimulus. Danger is defined as anything that threatens a person's physical, mental, emotional, and overall well-being. For you, that danger might be in the form of a family tragedy, work-life balance issues, relationships, self-esteem, economic issues, job loss, and the list goes on. When you are under stress, adrenaline is produced, triggering a fight-or-flight reaction. In modern society, the fight-or-flight reaction no longer looks like it did in the animal kingdom; instead, for many people it leads to either denying they are incapable of handling all that is on their plate and manically trying to attack everything at once, or shutting down completely. Respectively, either scenario can put us at risk for a mental and/or physical breakdown.

Research tells us that chronic stress disrupts nearly every system in the body. It can raise blood pressure, suppress the immune system, increase the risk of heart attack and stroke, contribute to infertility, and speed up the aging process. Long-term stress can even rewire the brain, leaving us more vulnerable to anxiety and depression.

Further, our body's stress hormone, cortisol, is secreted by the adrenal cortex in response to stress. Ongoing stress prolongs secretion, which over time has toxic effects on the body, causing negative consequences, including a severe weakening of the immune system and conditions such as hyperglycemia and obesity. The presence of cortisol, caused by long-term chronic stress, has been known to affect emotional, mental, and physical behavior, which can manifest as binge eating, panic attacks, nervous or physical breakdowns, random aches and pains, depression, heart disease, burnout, suicidal tendencies, and a variety of other problems.

Experiencing stress short-term and learning to react to it in more positive or proactive ways can motivate us to do our best.

But here's the interesting fact about stress: We can't ever eliminate it from our lives, nor should we want to. Experiencing stress short-term and learning to react to it in more positive or proactive ways can motivate us to do our best. Sometimes small doses of pressure and anxiety can encourage us to meet a deadline or get important things done. If we were never faced with the need to overcome challenges, we would never discover the pride of accomplishment we need to mature into confident and competent adults. Because of this, it isn't uncommon for people to experience Breakthroughs when under stress or as a result of something negative happening to them. It's when the pressure is on that we really find what we are made of. The trick is to react calmly to stress so that you know how to use those moments to your benefit. In the next chapter, we will learn how and why my 5 Living Principles of Well-Being are the perfect tool for learning to change negative reactions to stress.

Some stress is even necessary to help strengthen our body. Take lifting weights, even small ones. When you lift weights, you are stressing your muscles. The stress you put on your muscle actually causes the muscle to tear and as a response to this, the muscle compensates by increasing in strength and size as its fibers heal back together. The muscle is literally building itself up in reaction to stress. Now, if we can just do that for ourselves . . .

We can build ourselves up under stress using the secret we already know: you can't manage stress but you can give it a break.

Take a Break from Stress

Taking a break from stress helps you develop mental muscle and an emotional agility over time to cope better with stress. Continual efforts to manage stress signal the brain that this ongoing state is okay and creates a habit that might be masking its deleterious effects on your body. Learning to channel your reaction to stress differently helps to keep that mind-body connection positive, an integral part of the Anatomy of a Breakthrough. So, take a "stress break" and learn to give your body and mind the opportunity to recover and rebuild. Here are a few ideas I find work for me.

Take Five on Stress

1. Breathe Breath is life. Learning to breathe deeply and exhale slowly exercises control not just of the air passages, but helps improve physical and mental energy. Breathing helps you relax and find internal and external balance, stability, and freedom from the agitation that normally attends mental and physical pursuits. Breathing can help you learn to dispel unnecessary muscular tension and direct your energy to a more positive place.

The purposeful control of breathing in through your nose exercises and strengthens your diaphragm, filters the air, and promotes focus while conditioning and relaxing all your muscles. Inhale, taking in as much air as you possibly can, and hold it at the top of each breath for just a few seconds. Then exhale very slowly either through your nose or mouth, envisioning your lungs as if they were a deflating tire. You can learn to control your breath, improving on the depth and the length of time of each breath. The deeper the inhale and slower the release of air, the more relaxation you will experience.

Focusing on breath control as described above induces a positive meditative state as it limits unnecessary and unproductive distractions while promoting focus on the task at hand. Martial arts teach that the conscious awareness and control of one's breath helps focus mental and physical energy into the destructive kinetic power commonly associated with these Eastern practices. Conscious control with slow and rhythmic breaths *sifts out interfering thoughts, relaxes and readies the muscles, and funnels attention to a single task.* This process can be used to facilitate the early steps in the Anatomy of a Breakthrough (presence/mindfulness and awareness). Breath control is also easy to do, which is why it's such a convenient and strategically useful way to give stress a break and lay the groundwork to experience Break-throughs of your own.

2. Exercise

The same routine of regular exercise that helps prevent disease and builds muscles can also help you reduce stress by decreasing the production of stress hormones and counteracting your body's natural stress response. Exercise increases the production of endorphins, which are neurotransmitters produced by the pituitary gland that reduce pain and induce a sense of euphoria. The lasting effects of endorphins can sometimes continue as long as twelve hours. The classic example of this is what is commonly called *the runner's high.*

Exercise requires you to focus on the immediate task at hand. This process creates a meditative state with resulting energy and optimism. For instance, you shift your thinking away from the need to get the mail. You know it will still be in the mailbox when you come and get it later. Directing your concentration on the movements you are doing when participating in any form of exercise is what I call *Meditation in Motion.* You are using your physical body to center your mind onto something other than your daily tensions. Physical movement and the attention you have to give to the exercise cause you to redirect your thoughts away from other things in general, some of which might be negative. In doing so, your mind and mood are thereby improved.

Aside from the obvious benefits of exercise for weight control and overall health, exercise controls stress because it requires you to engage in something positive that is away from the situation or environment that is stressing you. Even ten minutes on a walk or on a stationary bike can be effective in taking your mind out of a negative state that prohibits Breakthroughs from happening.

A spontaneous decision to take a brisk walk around the office building in the middle of a flurry of e-mails, or right after a meeting goes awry can be a saving grace. A short walk can be calming and give you the ability to refocus—sometimes making you even more productive than when you first arrived that morning! This is because exercise of any kind increases circulation and especially blood flow to the brain. It also stimulates the metabolism and oxygenates the entire body, which boosts the performance you need when you are deeply engaged in something.

It is also helpful to look at exercise as a natural part of your day . . . like eating. You eat because it is enjoyable, or social, and provides fuel for what you want to do. Shift your approach to exercise by finding something you can do that is fun and also helps you feel good about yourself. Jump rope, take a bike ride, buddy up for a walk around the neighborhood, or just go outside with your kids for a game of catch or "hide and seek." You can start modestly, see and feel the benefits, and then add to it with SheaNetics.

If you look at exercise as a way to "take five" from stress and as part of a normal lifestyle—not strictly as a way to lose weight or worse, as "work"—you'll avoid defeating your good intentions by putting too much pressure on yourself. Without these self-induced expectations hovering over you, you will very likely find yourself exercising more often and longer than you originally planned. And anytime is a good time to start. Good exercise habits only produce good results. You'll feel energized, refocused, and ready (perhaps even with new solutions) for the challenges you took a break from in the first place.

3. Laugh Have you ever experienced a laugh that is so hearty it seems to affect you all over? It's the one that lasts a few minutes, gives you a tummy ache, and leads to tears streaming down your face. Sometimes you beg, "Please stop." Afterward, you are left feeling out of breath, exhausted, and in a totally different mood. *Oh, wow. That felt good. I really needed that.* Just writing about it here is causing me to smile!

We humans are designed to connect with each other through laughter. Laughter is an effective stress reducer, can relieve pain, and may even boost the immune system, making you less prone to developing colds and other infections.

Lifting yourself up with a chuckle helps you redirect your focus from what's bugging you, and, in turn, improves your disposition and mood so you can interact more meaningfully with others. Laughter is also a form of light exercise, clearing the breathing passage and filling the lungs and body with oxygen. In addition, it improves the function of blood vessels and increases blood flow, which can help protect against a heart attack and other car-diovascular problems.

When we laugh our bodies release a cocktail of hormones and chemicals that have a positive effect on our entire system, includ-ing the endorphins we previously mentioned. Positive emotions are associated with decreased production of the stress hormone cortisol, the damaging effects of which we also read about earlier. Laughter really is the "best medicine." Just ask Vince Vaughn, who makes us all laugh.

4. Music   If love gets credit for being the international language, then music must be hailed for its ability to universally express and move the essence of our humanity. Research has shown that music has a profound effect on our body and psyche.

Music with a strong beat can stimulate brainwaves to resonate in sync with the beat, causing greater concentration and more alert thinking; a slower beat promotes a calm, meditative state. Breathing and heart rate can also be altered depending on the type of music you listen to.

For instance, soft music has been shown to activate the relaxation response and can counteract or prevent the damaging effects of chronic stress. It has also been known to boost immunity, ease muscle tension, and more. Bringing music into your life is simple. With the proliferation of convenient media devices you can have the background music of your choice while driving, cooking, working on the computer, doing the laundry, cleaning the house, mowing the lawn, or doing other chores. There is music for any activity. My favorite music to listen to when I take a stress break or am teaching a class is one of my original SheaNetics CDs. It is a collection of universally appealing themes with just the right balance of melody and cadence, often over an ethereal background that soothes, energizes, and inspires your body, mind, and heart.

5. Think Positive

I know this is much easier said than done, and I am speaking from experience. But did you know pessimists are more likely to abandon their attempts to reach their goals? So instead, I try to focus on engaging in positive thinking and benefit from its power as hard as it may be at times. When you think negatively, you tend to wallow and linger within that state of negativity. It's a vibe that can suck you in and drown you like quicksand, but positivity throws you a tree branch to hold onto. Finding purpose in challenging situations and the silver lining in every cloud is how I have learned to respond. When it really becomes necessary, I try to keep my "pitty-pat-poor-me party" to sixty minutes, and then I pick myself up, dust myself off, and move on.

Finding purpose in challenging situations and the silver lining in every cloud is how I have learned to respond.

Shea's Breakthrough

My mother and my sister, Gail, were avid readers. In fact, when I was very little Gail would often read stories to me before going to bed. My mother was always doing crossword puzzles and playing Scrabble, and she passed on her passions to my sister and me. Mom taught us to play Scrabble, and we enjoyed that special time together. To this day, Gail and I play when she comes to visit, and when we get the board out and sit down to play we always say, "Mom is watching us and smiling." It was harder for me to learn to play than it was for my sister, and I thought it was because Gail was older. But, I also struggled with reading and word pronunciation in school. I wanted to read like my sister but found it difficult.

In school I was referred to as being a "slow learner." Hearing that was so hard, very hard. Any time you are *labeled* something, it is difficult to deal with—and it's particularly shattering for a child in elementary school, especially when you know it isn't true. I tried hard but knew there was some disconnect. A common theme reported home to my parents from my teachers was that I was not trying. This affected my self-esteem tremendously.

Back then, no one really knew what was going on, and they had no way of testing to pinpoint the problem. To add to the dilemma, my IQ test showed that I was "above average." This was in contrast to what my teacher seemed to see. She thought I was being lazy. To know that a person's perception of you could be so off base is disconcerting, and the more I thought about it, the greater my desire became to prove myself otherwise and the more pressure I felt. For instance, I would be so scared when the teacher called on me to read aloud in class. Little did anyone know how badly I wanted to please them and how much I wanted to learn. Faced by this challenge, I instead gained recognition and self-confidence in other ways by excelling in dance, gymnastics, and sports.

Some years after having school-aged children of my own, I began hearing about dyslexia from a conversation with a teacher. Children who are undiagnosed are often referred to as "slow learners," and because I recalled wearing that label, I began to wonder if perhaps I had dyslexia. After researching a bit more, I discovered that dyslexia can be a genetic condition. It wasn't long after that I put two and two together and learned that I, indeed, was dyslexic.

Although I thought I had moved on from those early labels

and the effect they had on my self-esteem, I felt a tremendous amount of freedom after I learned that my "slow learning" was actually because of a treatable condition; one we weren't equipped to diagnose or treat when I was a girl. It wasn't my fault that my sister was a better reader, and I wasn't stupid! I wanted to know everything, so I did research and discovered it has nothing to do with IQ or being lazy. In fact, people with dyslexia are notorious for being very hard workers.

I no longer felt alone and enjoyed relief in knowing I was not the only one with this genetic condition that often runs in families. My mother and father both had dyslexia, I learned. Moreover, I was in the good company of creative, successful, and intellectual people like Tom Cruise, Orlando Bloom, Cher, Walt Disney, Erin Brockovich, Thomas Edison, Nelson Rockefeller, Patrick Dempsey, Danny Glover, Sir Winston Churchill, Whoopi Goldberg, John F. Kennedy, and so many more. Their stories brought real inspiration and hope.

Positive thinking also made me realize that having an undiagnosed problem in childhood helped shape who I was to become in adulthood. Had I instead excelled in the areas with which I had struggled in school, I might not have turned my energy toward dance, gymnastic, athletics, and overall fitness—those disciplines about which I am passionate today. Having the struggles I did as a child actually made me a harder worker, enabling me to build a resilience and work ethic that I might not otherwise have had.

My Breakthrough came when many years later I learned to look back at these early experiences as positive gifts that led me to where, what, and who I am today. My perception changed. Challenges can be a catalyst for positive change; they can be motivational and even lead to a deeper sense of self-awareness and purpose. We may not always know exactly where the road is taking us, but lessons like these offer meaningful direction along the way.

Where stress is displaced, well-being emerges because it is not possible for the two to inhabit the same space. The future is uncertain and the past is already behind you, so please try to take a healthy break by focusing your thoughts on something or someone else and spend that time enjoyably. Be proactive in your pursuit of "stress breaks" and make them a regular part of your daily routine. You will regain energy, enjoy many Breakthroughs, find well-being, and increase the odds of living longer.

The Mother of All Stress Relievers: Meditation in Motion and Thought

I titled this chapter "Modern Meditation" because I wished to clarify what meditation has come to mean for many people and offer practical and effective ways to incorporate meditation into your life. Meditation is a powerful means to reduce stress by inviting calmness and clarity into your life. It is also a gateway to improving self-awareness and evaluation and to realizing things in ways you might not have been able to before—the essence of evoking Breakthroughs.

Upon hearing the word "meditate," many of us might conjure images of locking ourselves in a dark room and lighting candles while chanting or listening to mystic-sounding music. And, yes, while this can be one style of meditation, for many of us it is not an option that fits into our lives.

Meditation is another form of mindfulness, which we discussed in Chapter 3. It relieves the mind of oppressive or negative thinking, and in its place a more positive mental state can emerge.

A common misperception of many people is that the goal of meditation is to block out all thought, which is impossible because you are always thinking something. Instead, meditation is about establishing a different relationship with your thoughts, even if for a little while.

READER/CUSTOMER CARE SURVEY

We care about your opinions! Please take a moment to fill out our online Reader Survey at **http://survey.hcibooks.com.**

As a **"THANK YOU"** you will receive a **VALUABLE INSTANT COUPON** towards future book purchases

as well as a **SPECIAL GIFT** available only online! Or, you may mail this card back to us.

(PLEASE PRINT IN ALL CAPS)

First Name _____ MI. _____ Last Name _____

Address _____ City _____

State _____ Zip _____ Email _____

1. Gender
- ❑ Female   ❑ Male

2. Age
- ❑ 8 or younger
- ❑ 9-12   ❑ 13-16
- ❑ 17-20   ❑ 21-30
- ❑ 31+

3. Did you receive this book as a gift?
- ❑ Yes   ❑ No

4. Annual Household Income
- ❑ under $25,000
- ❑ $25,000 - $34,999
- ❑ $35,000 - $49,999
- ❑ $50,000 - $74,999
- ❑ over $75,000

5. What are the ages of the children living in your house?
- ❑ 0 - 14   ❑ 15+

6. Marital Status
- ❑ Single
- ❑ Married
- ❑ Divorced
- ❑ Widowed

7. How did you find out about the book?
(please choose one)
- ❑ Recommendation
- ❑ Store Display
- ❑ Online
- ❑ Catalog/Mailing
- ❑ Interview/Review

8. Where do you usually buy books?
(please choose one)
- ❑ Bookstore
- ❑ Online
- ❑ Book Club/Mail Order
- ❑ Price Club (Sam's Club, Costco's, etc.)
- ❑ Retail Store (Target, Wal-Mart, etc.)

9. What subject do you enjoy reading about the most?
(please choose one)
- ❑ Parenting/Family
- ❑ Relationships
- ❑ Recovery/Addictions
- ❑ Health/Nutrition
- ❑ Christianity
- ❑ Spirituality/Inspiration
- ❑ Business Self-help
- ❑ Women's Issues
- ❑ Sports

10. What attracts you most to a book?
(please choose one)
- ❑ Title
- ❑ Cover Design
- ❑ Author
- ❑ Content

FOLD HERE

Comments

You are training yourself to place your attention when and where you want it—Directed Concentration. To that end, meditation is a practice of concentrated focus upon a sound, object, visualization, the breath, or movement in order to increase awareness of the present moment. This contemplative state can be induced through physical (exercise) and/or mental effort, which narrows and redirects activity or thought in a single direction or toward a specific purpose, from "point A" to "point B."

A common misperception of many people is that the goal of meditation is to block out all thought, which is impossible because you are always thinking something.

Remember the examples in "Take Five on Stress"? Those suggestions were simple tools to physically and/or mentally assist you in redirecting your concentration and to help you refocus from negative to positive things. So, really engaging and focusing on any activity that brings you joy, produces a chemical reaction in your body, and takes you out of the stressful moment (even for a short period) is a form of meditation. When you make a conscious effort of self-directed focus, you can put yourself in a meditative state.

Meditation can be achieved through either a physical or mental "trigger" or a combination of both, which I call "Meditation in Motion (physical) and Thought (mental)." *Meditation in Motion* means you achieve mental concentration through the body's effort in movement, as described in the discussion above on exercise. Again, because you are using your physical body to center your mind on something other than your daily tensions, you improve your state of mind and your mood through movement. The very act of you directing your concentration on the movement or sequence you are doing becomes, in itself, meditative.

The very act of you directing your concentration on the movement or sequence you are doing becomes, in itself, meditative.

Similarly, *Meditation in Thought* means you use your mind to consciously channel your thought to exclude distractions, particularly ones that are causing you stress, and direct and redirect your thinking (and mood) in a more productive and peaceful direction. This can be achieved through repeating a word or phrase, or through engaging in positive thinking and/or visualization.

We can reduce stress through meditation and have seen how we can achieve a less anxious state in a number of ways. But once there, how do we fully reap its benefits? How do we unlock the Anatomy of a Breakthrough and fully utilize its potential? It is through The 5 Living

Principles of Well-Being. They are words you can repeat to yourself, concepts that help you replace negativity with positivity, and they are very powerful. The 5 Living Principles are beacons of light that can instantly remove you from moments of stress and lead you to act and react in healthier and more rewarding ways.

If you look closely at the Anatomy of a Breakthrough you will see that it is a process comprised of beautiful and complex pieces that fit together like a mosaic—delicately and purposefully. Breakthroughs require calmness and clarity, mindfulness and awareness, a positive mind-body connection, and the release of stress that might interfere with that connection. Up to this point, we have discussed these various aspects separately. It's time to bring these pieces together, because as each one adheres to the next, only then do we set the conditions for real lasting change.

But how do we begin to create our mosaic? What is the glue that makes it all come—and stay—together? The answer lies within a new code for living, within a safe place for self-reflection and personal change . . . within The 5 Living Principles of Well-Being.

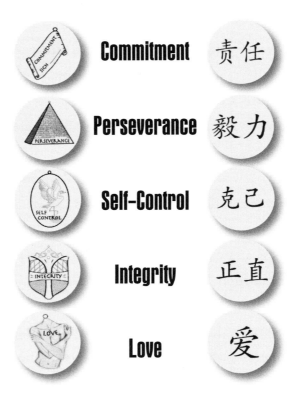

The 5 Living Principles of Well-Being are your foundation and positive reinforcement to reduce stress, help you make better choices, and improve the overall quality of your life and the lives of those around you. Let's take a look at how each Principle brings meaning into your life.

CHAPTER FIVE

The 5 Living Principles of Well-Being

The Anchor Philosophy for All You Do

> *"Go confidently in the direction*
> *of your dreams. Live the life*
> *you have imagined."*
>
> —Henry David Thoreau

Life may feel at times like a series of struggles, and as we've discussed, how we respond to them leaves us feeling up or down, powerful or weak, invincible or vulnerable. This seesaw ride contributes to the chipping away of our sense of balance and self-worth. Ultimately for each of us, well-being is our goal, but we find it difficult to achieve because we lack the control over our circumstances, our reactions to them, and even our very will.

Philosophy from that of Plato to Marcus Aurelius to Nietzsche to Kant was born out of humans' desire to make sense of things, to find meaning where there was thought to be none, and to help set priorities by which to live. The goal, whether you follow their philosophies or find fault with their questions and musings, is to gain a sense of control in a complex, chaotic world.

One of my personal philosophies is the only aspect of life over which you have control is yourself and how you react to what happens to you.

While many "official" philosophies for living emerged from pioneers as early as the Classical Era, today people of every walk of life might say they have a "philosophy of life." For some people it may be "to be a good person"; to reject material things; to "do unto others as you would have done unto you"; or to "work hard/play hard." Whatever the philosophy, it is a personal choice and acts as a guide and a reminder of what's important to you, and, most important, helps you stay on track when you feel you may be heading astray.

One of my personal philosophies is the *only aspect of life over which you have control is yourself and how you react to what happens to you.* What's your personal philosophy? Take a minute or two or several more here, and write down some philosophies you either already live by, or would like to:

_____

_____

_____

_____

_____

_____

_____

_____

How do you feel? Perhaps you feel more grounded or directed in a way that you haven't felt before. By recording your life philosophies, your journey in life may feel more defined, because you have created tools—on your own terms—to help guide you to live in a way that reflects who you truly are. When you feel down or defeated, stressed or alienated, turning to your life philosophies can act as a reminder that you are doing the best you can and assist you in discovering the power within you to defeat whatever it is that is before you.

The 5 Living Principles of Well-Being were derived from my personal need to find a way to articulate the code by which I want to live. They act as a philosophy for living, tools to help control my reaction to negative things, and transitory guides that enable me to address situations better by dissipating the stress and anxiety that, at times, cloud my better judgment.

The 5 Living Principles are transformative; they help redirect your present state of mind and evoke mindfulness of the present moment, also referred to as a meditative state. However, let me be clear: this alone will not bring on a Breakthrough. Thinking about the Principles may bring on presence of mind, but how you use them is what empowers Breakthroughs. The Principles guide you to a healthier lifestyle and way of thinking, they help you make better choices, inspire you to be a kinder and more thoughtful individual, and much more.

The Principles lead you into a meditative state, and once there you are able to refocus and examine the what, how, who, and when. Your concentration can bring clarity to confirm, or not, that what you are considering needs change, or not.

But before we learn how to apply The 5 Living Principles of Well-Being to each area of your life—from defeating stress and gaining health and vitality, to eating well and exercising more, to feeling younger and looking vibrant and having better self-esteem for the rest of your life—first let me reintroduce to you The 5 Living Principles of Well-Being:

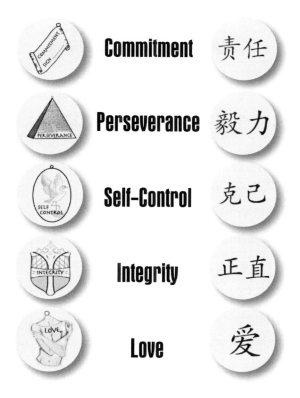

Each of The 5 Living Principles of Well-Being is designed to bring a unique benefit and level of meaning into your life. Used individually or collectively, they will create positive energy in any situation, anywhere, and at any time. They are *Meditation in Thought,* and will invite Breakthroughs into your life.

Commitment

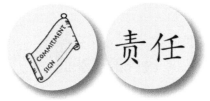

Commitment is a promise to do something, whether it is to work out, seek better health, find a new job, or be a better person. The *Scroll* represents a binding contract you have signed to honor your promise.

It's so easy to put yourself last. In fact, most of us, especially women, do. For some reason it is easier to keep promises to others. We don't want to let anyone down, but in reality, the act of ignoring what we pledge to ourselves induces a neglect that can be devastating to the health of our minds and bodies. You would never tell your children you will pick them up from school at a certain time and not show up. But when it comes to the things you planned for yourself—that overdue haircut, trying out that new pilates class at the gym, going back to school—you don't give a second thought to breaking that commitment to yourself. A promise is, and should be at all times, a commitment—period.

It can be as simple as setting and keeping a regular time to work out or attend a class. Certainly, without this dedication or self-discipline there can be no physical improvement. Keeping to a schedule is critical to the efficient and effective management of our daily activities and to the timely completion of tasks. Success is not an accident, but the result of a well-executed plan.

Commitment is the first Principle for good reason. Wanting something for yourself is not the same as promising it to yourself. You may want to be in great shape or want to have a better job but you won't begin to get there unless, and until, you make the promise to yourself.

Making a commitment to achieving better health gets you off the couch and on the go. Aspiring to higher levels of individual growth and accomplishment, whether personal or careerwise, takes a commitment to following your dream, maybe by networking with friends, working with management, or getting online to search for that new job or curriculum. You begin to *live* when you make a pledge to do something good for yourself. It's like taking a giant leap—a leap of faith in you!

A True Story of **Commitment**

Gregory is married with three children. He is even-tempered, faithful to his family, hard working. He is also handy; if you need help with fixing or building something he will be there without expecting anything in return. One day we were talking and he confided in me that his wife, who is a loving, sweet, and involved mother, recently gave him an ultimatum. While he is a good provider, and she, a great mom, she felt frustrated by an emotional distance she believed he had created between himself and her and the kids. In nothing less than black-and-white terms, she told Gregory to either open up more to her and the kids, essentially putting in the same hard work into his family life that he does his work life, or she would file for divorce.

The entire family needed more interaction and affection from him, and Gregory wanted to understand why he struggled to show his love. He sought answers within himself and came to believe that his coming from a divorced family, where there was little to no affection and where a focus on work life prevailed, had contributed to him continuing a cycle that was destined to destroy his own family.

Gregory wanted to turn things around, and he said to me that he first needed to learn to love himself—to not let the lack of love he felt in childhood overbear his emotions and actions in adulthood. After searching and practicing the Principle of Commitment, which helped him dedicate himself to saving his family and creating a fulfilling family life, he realized he was a caring and good person who very much believed that family should always come first.

Gregory told me that in order to really change his situation and not lose his family he needed to Commit to making immediate and critical lifestyle changes. Commitment is contagious, so once he ignited the Principle of Commitment and put it to use, it was almost impossible to reverse its powerful force. Gregory is now Committed to keeping what he's come to know he loves and cherishes most in life—his wife and children—despite the fact that the same wasn't bestowed upon him growing up. Commitment led Gregory to a Breakthrough—he didn't have to continue a cycle of hurt and loss. His decision to Commit was his alone and helped him assess his situation clearly and find the strength and courage to make real changes in his life and the life of his family.

Unfortunately, for so many of us, making necessary changes only occurs to us when we are near disaster, or until we are threatened with an ultimatum or intervention that startles us into evoking action. The Principle of Commitment can help us take responsibility for what needs to be done—when we are ready—without regret or shame.

Perseverance

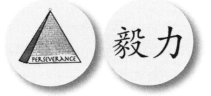

Perseverance is the perpetual belief that if I try I will succeed. The *Pyramid* reminds us that the pathway to well-being is continuous, and you build toward your goal one solid step at a time.

Something as simple as curiosity might bring you to a new endeavor, but perseverance is what helps you do it and keep at it. The phrase *Rome wasn't built in a day* acknowledges that things worth doing take time. To reach higher levels in your life, achieve any goal you set for yourself, or feel emotionally better means staying motivated and in relentless pursuit. Your eye should always be on the prize, but incorporating the Principle of Perseverance into your daily living can help you maintain the physical and emotional energy it takes to do so.

Getting dressed and showing up to work out is more than half the battle, but following through by making your workouts habitual takes perseverance. You have choices. Many students new to physical training find that the first several weeks of any regular exercise are the most challenging. Inevitably, they find that the body grows stronger and adds definition as it progresses through this period. "Perseverance pays off," just as *The Little Engine That Could* discovered. Continuing to give life to this Principle is what keeps you training.

It's no different when training for mental pursuits. Once you Commit to live in pursuit of your dreams, no matter the obstacles, remind yourself to always stay the course amidst the challenges. It will make you a powerful force with which to contend.

Perseverance encourages you to stay engaged. Success is yours if you want it, but you can't get it unless you get off the couch and into the game. The point to be remembered was immortalized by Satchel Paige in his popular saying about baseball, "You win a few, you lose a few. Some get rained out. But you got to dress for all of them." You will never attain your goal unless you persist in making the effort. So "suit up."

A True Story of **Perseverance**

As a child, Miriam was told she was too fat. Growing up, she wanted to lose weight but found it hard to avoid junk food, especially her favorites—soda, candy, potato chips, and dip. Try as she did, she just couldn't stick to a healthy diet. Miriam was raised by her grandparents, who loved her and took care of her, but also indulged her. In their minds, it was easier to let Miriam have what she wanted, and so she was left with no guidance to help her lose weight. Being excessively overweight creates obvious health issues, but the mental abuse that it projects onto those who grapple with obesity can cause deep damage.

In her midtwenties and with the help of her best friend, who exercised regularly and ate a more balanced diet, Miriam began to understand what it takes to shed pounds. She started exercising, building up to a commendable three times a week for forty-five minutes; she gave up soda and added more fruits and vegetables to her diet. The Principle of Perseverance was what it took to get her to stay on track and feel so much better about herself.

Miriam shared with me that she sometimes still feels like the "too fat" little girl but realizes that's not who she is today. Hurtful labels given to anyone can destroy confidence and keep us from moving forward to a more positive and productive life. You just need to look at yourself in the mirror and say, "That label is not who I am now." The act of doing that alone is Perseverance, as you consciously decide to overcome your past, accept your flaws, and work through your doubts so you can achieve whatever it is you desire.

Self-Control

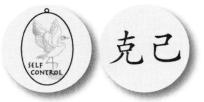

Self-Control is the realization that you are responsible for everything you do. When you stop to think about it, how you react to the events happening in your life is the only outcome of any event you can consciously determine. The *Crane*, as it stands on one leg, represents the balance and grace to be attained in life when you have found a way to control your emotions. Control your emotions, and your body will follow.

The Crane, as it stands on one leg, represents the balance and grace to be attained in life when you have found a way to control your emotions.

For instance, this Principle suggests that during a workout you have a sense of what your body is doing and the degree of your mental involvement and response. Using this self-awareness allows you to make the decision of whether to hold a stretch or pose a bit longer, listen to the instructor, or look out the window. What *you* choose will affect the quality of your experience, what you learn, and whether or not you make positive contributions to your workout.

This is especially true in life. Possessing an even temperament in stressful situations is of obvious personal benefit, but probably one of the most difficult things to achieve. Wouldn't it feel good to speed up next to that driver who just cut you off, roll down your window, and scream at the top of your lungs while honking your horn? . . . But does it *really* feel good? After all is said and done, and the driver says a few choice words back and you almost risk the lives of innocent people on the road, have you really accomplished anything? Do you really feel . . . good? Your blood is boiling, your heart is racing, you are out of the moment, and your awareness remains fixated on the jerk in the car.

This is no condition for a Breakthrough, but the Principle of Self-Control is here to help you find sanity in situations that test your patience and willpower when you least expect it. Turning on the radio, taking a deep breath (literally), or consciously tuning into this Principle by saying it out loud—any or all of these would be healthier choices. A Breakthrough will occur: the feeling that at first you are captive to your emotions, and then discovering you really have other alternatives that are far more beneficial.

Rudyard Kipling's inspirational poem "If—" says it best: "If you can keep your head when all about you are losing theirs . . . Yours is the Earth and everything that's in it. . . . "

Self-Control is about choice. Let's say your flight is canceled, your teenager stays out after curfew, your overbearing relative from out of state suddenly shows up at your front door, or the promotion you expected goes to someone else. What actions and words would you choose to handle these situations? When your best friends show up at the house hours late to a dinner party you planned months in advance, saying, "Sorry we got a late start," can you simply smile and say, "Great . . . you're just in time for dessert"?

How do you handle stress, anxiety, or frustration? Self-Control reminds you that your reaction is *your* choice, and being ever aware of this Principle is an important step in giving yourself the gift of inner strength necessary to respond with greater dignity and wisdom.

A True Story of **Self-Control**

Ali loved to go shopping. She had more clothes than anyone I had ever known. I can remember thinking, *How can she afford to spend so much money on clothes?* One day her husband mentioned that her addictive spending was going to cost them their marriage and home. Whenever I approached the subject of her spending, she would simply say that her husband makes good money and wants her to look her best.

It wasn't too soon after that Ali's husband dropped a bomb and served her divorce papers. They had two wonderful children together, who didn't want to see their parents separate. They loved both parents and had been the recipients of Ali's generosity—when she went shopping, she always bought clothes for the entire family. It was something she loved to do, but her children realized she had become excessive about her habit and agreed their father could not afford to continue to let their mother spend all of their money.

Ali's husband agreed that if she went to counseling, which he had begged her to do for years, he would give their marriage another try. She agreed, and along her way to self-discovery she learned her spending was a coping mechanism that was the result of underlying issues she had never really faced. As a child she was locked in her bedroom for hours and many times without something to eat. She was made to wear the same clothes to school every day until she was old enough to get a job and buy her own clothes. At age twenty-two, her life changed when both of her parents were killed suddenly in an automobile accident, and because she was an only child, she inherited their house and money. It wasn't long before she began to compensate for her feelings of deprivation and loss. Her Self-Control was out of control as she used shopping to fill voids she had buried deep down.

Predictably, as Ali compensated for her emotional emptiness through reckless spending, her credit card debt mounted precipitously. However, at age twenty-six she was lucky enough to meet her future husband-to-be who generously paid off her credit card and helped her sell the house. At the time he attributed her monetary situation and spending habits to the tragedy of losing her parents at an early age and not having the necessary financial maturity. However, over time he clearly had learned it was not that simple.

"Getting well" for Ali will be a long, arduous process, but one that can also be extremely rewarding. The healing began when she acknowledged her past and the effect it had on her. She had a number of issues and memories to deal with, but she also had to take responsibility for her actions and decide what she would do in the future. Analysis of her behavior led her to realize she was responding to deep-seated issues and unresolved needs. Her Breakthrough occurred when she admitted her need to have and to exert Self-Control. For her it will take tremendous effort and be something she has to work at every day.

Integrity

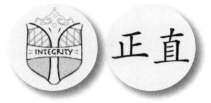

Integrity does not examine the result—only the effort made. It is the level of honesty in the quality of effort you give to the execution of whatever you strive to do. The *Shield* represents trustworthiness and your steadfast adherence to a strict code of moral and ethical behavior.

The self-knowledge of always being engaged to the best of your ability gives you pride and confidence. You see this in children. When children are excited about doing something, they give it their best effort with no holding back. Often it takes more than one try, but the effort is always the maximum. Children do not see barriers. The simple act of doing is as fulfilling as the pride resulting from their accomplishment.

Rediscover and bring forth your "inner child." The honesty applied to your physical and/or emotional training is what projects you to a higher plane of accomplishment. At any age you have limitations, but as long as you are aware of them, that awareness helps you to remain active. Practicing the Principle of Integrity allows you to express yourself completely and at increasing levels of effort. You can learn for yourself what a great spirit you have inside and the sense of pride that comes with that discovery.

Your body is a wonderful machine and your mind a magnificent instrument, but without further challenge you plateau and even decline in capability. Investing greater effort is necessary to grow or even maintain these gifts. Showing Integrity is telling yourself, *I can't do it today, but I'll keep trying.* Say to yourself every day, *I am gong to try to do the best stretch, deepest bend, or highest leg lift I can do. I will rock this presentation. I will make this a win-win deal.* Most important is the spirit with which you attempt each action. Take each as it comes, but always give it your best effort. Remember, it all doesn't have to be done at once.

There is no finer compliment in life than being known as an individual of Integrity. A reputation for Integrity flows from a history of fairness with others. One fair act can establish your trustworthiness. For example, giving credit to someone else who deserves it, standing up for what you believe, allowing others to be heard, doing the right thing when there is no one else around to see it. Opportunities like these exist for us every day.

This Principle of Integrity encourages you to take the high road. It takes great character to bring this kind of honest effort to all of your engagements and undertakings. However, it suggests to others an exceptional degree of truthfulness in your personal dealings and relationships. You will be appreciated, admired, and rewarded with a well-deserved sense of pride.

A True Story of **Integrity**

I was attending an outdoor concert some time ago with close friends and thousands of others. Moving through the crowds amidst the sea of people in lawn chairs, Chris, one of our group and a really good guy, saw a one-hundred-dollar bill on the ground. He picked it up and instinctively began to ask everyone around us if they had dropped the bill. A nearby group spoke up, instantly claiming it. As Chris approached them with bill in hand, they laughed and thanked him and then asked, "Did you know this is fake?"

"No, I can't see that well," he answered.

As we walked away we heard them say, "Now, *there's* an honest man."

> Chris drew satisfaction from knowing he'd done the right thing, but it was surpassed by our realization that through his honest actions, he gave hope to a group of people who had perhaps become a bit too cynical about life. His simple yet honorable act had an unintended benefit by demonstrating there are still people with Integrity who believe in making this world a fair and honest one. Hopefully, they were inspired to pay it forward.

Love

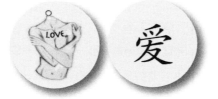

Love is openness and respect for yourself, for others, and for life itself. It is the willingness to explore and interact with people, to listen, learn, share, and to *always set the best example possible*. The *Crossed Arms* symbolize universal love.

Love is universal. It takes so many different forms it is possible to feel its effects in every aspect of our lives. Love is also a very special gift: from one spouse to another, from a mother and father to their child, or from one friend to another. It's also there in a Good Samaritan's selfless kindness toward a stranger or even a soldier's sacrifice for his or her country. Love is energy—it is the purpose of life. Love is what makes us whole and keeps our hearts beating and alive.

Pause to appreciate the people in your life, the causes that have meaning to you, and the things that add value to your life and you can feel the richness of living. Allow yourself to be humbled by the kind acts of others and the care shown to you, and it adds to the meaning to be learned from any experience. It is of fundamental importance, too, for you to embrace a Love of yourself as well, and with it comes peace, confidence, and the sense that everything about you is aligned. Love emanates from within and is what enables us to meaningfully connect with others. It is the critical component to the proper functioning of the social fabric of our lives and completes our existence.

Pause to appreciate the people in your life, the causes that have meaning to you, and the things that add value to your life and you can feel the richness of living.

When we are first conceived, the first cell is the beginning of a heart. The brain may direct each beat, but we still feel the heart as the real center of our being and the well from which all of our caring and love comes. Self-love is truly the greatest gift we can give ourselves and others, as Gregory learned in the earlier story. Without loving himself first and acknowledging that he deserved the Love of others because of his worth, he would not have been able to make the Commitment to show Love to his wife and children.

The Principle of Love is about loving yourself and loving others enough to set the right example. It's do as I do. This may be simple to express, but sometimes difficult to accomplish. True Love calls for personal sacrifice. Show tolerance for others, their ideas, methods of expression, and beliefs. Share your enthusiasm for something, continue your journey of personal development, and spark the same desire in others. Be gentle with the hearts of others, and, if not returned, try to understand their shortcomings, but do not enable them.

The Principle of Love is tied closely with the act of forgiveness, because Love should be unconditional. When you place no conditions on your feeling for others, it is easier to forgive, which is one of the most freeing acts a human can exercise.

Shea's Breakthrough

When the kids were young we had a small Maltese dog we named Vladimir. Very sadly, one Halloween night she ran out of the house and into the street and got hit by a car. Shortly thereafter, we bought another Maltese and named him Varo. Unfortunately, he did not have the loving disposition that Vladimir had. In fact, he bit our next-door neighbor and snapped at all of us, growling to leave him alone. We had to always be on guard as he would frequently rush outside through an opened door, and we would have to go and find him.

I became very frustrated over the dog and threatened a number of times to give him away. So after four years I psyched myself up, telling myself that the kids would get over it and it really was not a big deal. Meanwhile, I had not considered how losing Varo might affect all of my children, especially my middle daughter, Valeri, because she spent the most time with him and considered him her dog. So I gave the dog away and when the kids came home from school I told them that Varo had run away. Of course they searched for him, but he was nowhere to be found. I started to feel this deep sickness inside that kept nagging at me. Little did I know this was only the beginning of what I would end up feeling. Several months later the kids started questioning me, asking if he had actually run away or if I had given him away. I wasn't ready to fall on my sword quite yet. So of course, I stuck to my story but later learned that this was not the last we would talk about it.

About four months later I thought if we bought another dog it would ease matters and all would be forgotten. So we bought a little brown Chihuahua and named her Vanidice ("Vanny" for short). Valeri picked her out of the litter, but because my mom was home all of the time, Vanny spent more time with Jeanette and slept with her every night. Nonetheless, the topic of Varo kept coming up over the years and Valeri would continue to remind me, "You know, Mom, Varo was very important to me because I felt he was the only thing that was really mine." So over the years the guilt, the embarrassment, and the realization of the pain and distrust I had caused never left my mind or my heart. At the time when I made the decision to give Varo away I was not able to clearly assess the ripple effects or the consequences and pain this decision would have on all of us. I wanted desperately to tell the truth, to be honest about what had really happened, but felt that the kids wouldn't understand and would not forgive me. I didn't feel I had a "safe space" in which to go!

Time passed, but one day when Valeri was home with me alone and we were talking she said, "Mom, I want to talk to you about Varo." Instantly, my heart sank. She continued to say, "Mom, I want to provide a *safe space* for you, and I'm sorry that I didn't do this until now, so that you could come to me and tell me the truth. . . . But I want to know the truth and put this behind us."

I can remember looking at my daughter and saying, "I love you with all my heart and I thank you for being you. I've wanted to tell you the truth for so long but didn't know how to, especially after all this time." So I told her the truth, and we sat and talked for a while. We hugged, we cried, and it made me think about the "safe space" scenario and the importance of what it can do, and the opportunities it can provide for everyone. I know I am not the only person who ever wanted to say something or address a problem but didn't feel safe doing so. For most people, if they don't feel safe, they probably won't say something.

It taught me the importance of providing a "safe space," opening the door for someone to say, "I'm sorry." It doesn't mean you condone their actions or in any way agree with what they did or said. But acknowledging that we are all human, we all are vulnerable and make mistakes, we all need to be forgiven for something, and we all need to have the opportunity to move on with our lives, is the ultimate expression of Love.

My daughter gave me an invitation to "Breakthrough." It was a powerful lesson about love and forgiveness. I truly learned that actions have consequences, and the importance of accepting responsibility for our actions. This isn't something new, but like many things in life, we don't learn our lessons until it happens to us. Do not take these matters lightly. Think thoroughly before you take action. It also might be the right time to provide a "safe space" or to take matters into your hands and address something that has lingered way to long. Your decisions are still your own but as you reason through them, remember: if your mind is open and your heart is loving, it will bring peace to you and to others.

The 5 Living Principles of Well-Being are the anchor philosophy for all you do. When your actions are put into the context of one or more of the Principles, it helps you focus on what is before you and to be more in the moment . . . to not just experience life, but to experience the experience of life. It puts what you do into a meaningful context, whether the benefit is immediate or to be realized in the future. The Principles help you initiate presence of mind, increase awareness, and exert a positive and objective influence as you evaluate matters. When we embrace the Principles as both guide and inspiration, the emphasis is placed on the process, not the conclusion. However, the individual actions that do flow from calling upon them become part of a greater goal that is to live with purpose and meaning. This is really learning to live life well, and it brings its own rewards.

Now that we have explored each of The 5 Living Principles of Well-Being as the anchor philosophy for all we do, we can now learn how to apply the Principles to achieve the things we wish for in life. But, first, what is on *your* wish list?

WHAT'S ON YOUR WISH LIST?

One of the crucial steps in Breakthroughs is taking stock of your life's wish list. By examining both old and new desires, goals, and daydreams, you can decide what's doable, how to achieve it, what you've actually already achieved, and what's not as important to you today as it once was. When you do these things, you are exercising the first and second steps in the Anatomy of a Breakthrough—deciding to be in the moment and becoming aware. Once you complete those steps your mind is refocused and set to a new task. You now can assess where you want to go and the best way to go about getting there—and you will be one step closer to a Breakthrough.

While you are in the moment, do you wish . . .?

- I wish I felt happy
- I wish I had more time
- I wish I felt like I had more control over my life
- I wish I had more energy
- I wish I could lose weight
- I wish I could eat healthier
- I wish I felt like working out
- I wish I could sleep better
- I wish I were fit
- I wish I weren't so nervous
- I wish I looked like I did ten years ago

If any of these thoughts or something similar has crossed your mind, it could be that what you're really saying is, "I want to feel good about my life and myself." Take a minute now and list your wishes below. Be sure to remember old dreams that still tug on your heart, or things you sometimes only daydream about. Everything counts here, so really search every corner of your mind, heart, and soul.

I Wish: _____

_____

_____

_____

_____

How Long Have I Had This Wish? _____

_____

What's Holding Me Back? _____

_____

_____

_____

I Wish: _____

_____

_____

_____

_____

_____

How Long Have I Had This Wish? _____

_____

What's Holding Me Back? _____

_____

_____

I Wish: _____

_____

_____

_____

_____

_____

How Long Have I Had This Wish? _____

_____

What's Holding Me Back? _____

_____

_____

Don't be overwhelmed with the need to do everything at once and end up doing nothing, allowing self-doubt to win and take control of your destination. Instead, tell yourself, *I know I can't do it all today . . . but I can start with one wish, along with The 5 Living Principles, to rebuild my life and be a better role model for myself and those I love.*

Get started by making a **Commitment. Perseverance** will keep you on your journey with **Integrity** as your compass. Don't hesitate—create a plan, step forward, and have fun. Be proactive in whatever you do. Don't stop there! Once you experience the success of your first wish continue down the list . . . one at a time. Find the **Self-Control** you may temporarily let slip away, and use the same action plan to fulfill all your wishes. Remember always to **Love** yourself through it all.

CHAPTER SIX

Putting The 5 Living Principles of Well-Being to Work in Your Life

SheaNetics in Action

"Life is a journey, not a destination."

—Ralph Waldo Emerson

In The 5 Living Principles of Well-Being, I have found a fundamentally simple and motivational code for living that helps infuse my life with positivity, well-being, and Breakthroughs. The Principles are the inspirational guide for all I do, and now they will be for you too!

By making the Principles part of your daily life, you focus on creating positive energy, and thereby create a mental and physical state that allows you to be open to experiencing Breakthroughs.

This may be a time in your life when you feel you are at a crossroads. In seeking out this book, you have already proven to yourself that you are ready to take greater stock of where you are in your life— and a candid look at where you would like to go from here. Whether you are searching for answers to help you make more informed and healthier decisions or are seeking deeper purpose and meaning in all that you do, you are now at a point in your life where you are experienced enough to appreciate the benefits that come from overcoming the obstacles before you.

If experiencing Breakthroughs is not a familiar part of your life, perhaps you have lacked effective tools to help you properly open up and embrace their power. Fear, complacency, comfort, or disinterest may be what is holding you back, but no longer.

The biggest Breakthrough of all is the ability to live The 5 Living Principles of Well-Being so they can allow you to be open to Breakthroughs that happen on a day-to-day basis. This is my biggest wish for you, so that you can live a clearer, more defined life and be better equipped to deal with your challenges with increased focus and reasoning and less emotion. To—in the face of doubt, stress, and confusion—respond with grace, self-assuredness, boldness, and dignity. To make progress in ways you have only dreamed of and get the results you know deep down you deserve. With The 5 Living Principles of Well-Being at your side, anything is possible. Now let's learn by example how to put them to work in your life.

I believe we are all here to learn certain lessons, and the sooner we can begin conquering the challenges that hold us back, the sooner we can move on to a more fulfilling and loving life. Most of us are at one time or another, dealing (or trying to cope) with complicated issues that keep us spinning our wheels, in a state of self-doubt, or far away from experiencing Breakthroughs. I call these issues the Big Four, and for women especially, they are most pervasive. The Big Four, as I see them, include: self-esteem, health and fitness, work-life balance, and aging.

I believe we are all here to learn certain lessons, and the sooner we can begin conquering the challenges that hold us back, the sooner we can move on to a more fulfilling and loving life.

These Big Four have, at one point and in some form, affected us or someone we love (or both). In order to defeat them, we must honestly assess our reaction to them and the affect they are having on us. This means admitting some of our own shortcomings, which is a vital part of having life-enhancing revelations. We must be willing to evaluate ourselves honestly and not allow fear and vulnerability to sabotage our progress.

Meet Corrine: Self-Esteem

After eighteen years working for an ad agency, the work had become mundane. It wasn't always boring and predictable; admittedly at one time it had been fun. Corrine thought she would simply retire there, in the same department she had always worked in: accounts receivable. She was fully vested and her stock options were promising (if and when the market turned around), so while the work had become a bland routine, she felt seduced into finishing out her career there and to maxing out on her benefits. *In this climate, security is all that matters*, she'd tell herself.

Corrine was able to keep from going crazy over the grind of what she, with a "tongue-in-cheek" respect, would refer to as "corporate predictability" and "bureaucratic sensibility," because she had an outlet—cake pops. She often made them herself in her spare time. They were cake on a stick, round and beautifully decorated, thanks to the fondant class she took at her local bakery on Saturday mornings.

They were all the rage, and she was actually able to sell a few to friends and friends of friends who were looking for unique favor items for birthday parties or school functions.

With each pop she created, Corrine found herself engaged and excited. *Wouldn't it be terrific to do this full time!*

Two weeks and two days after she marked her eighteenth year at the agency, her manager called her in. She suspected something, as there were rumors of downsizing as new accounts dwindled and the entire advertising industry changed, thanks to the invention of DVR and TiVo. But somehow she thought they would get rid of the support staff first or, with business being off, maybe a few of the higher-ups whose big base salaries might now be considered a fiscal road bump. It never dawned on her that she'd go first.

When her manager broke the bad news, Corrine found herself a little frozen in place. It was a shock, and she struggled to keep her composure. There was also injury added to the sting of being let go. Eighteen years just didn't seem to matter. It was a short conversation, and she left swiftly, just like you see in the movies, except she had two guards escort her out of the building. As she closed the door to her car, the blood was rushing straight to her head and the back of her neck began to ache. She didn't dare turn the key in the ignition. She feared she would faint behind the wheel and called her girlfriend to come and pick her up.

"I've been fired, Jackie. Fired! Downsized. Whatever it's called, they just let me go. Please come get me," she said, her voice shaking.

Corinne immediately went into panic mode. She couldn't survive on the three-month severance the agency "so kindly" gave her, and she was still too young to begin to draw on her retirement. Nor did she want to borrow against it. Even if she could get past her own stigma about unemployment compensation, it just was not going to be enough. She thought again, *Security is everything.*

Corrine spent the next two months pounding the pavement, which today translates into searching the Internet, calling and e-mailing old contacts, and even putting out a new status on her Facebook page: "Unemployed and Looking."

One afternoon, defeated and full of tears, Corrine called Jackie to come over and keep her company.

"When was the last time you left the house, Corrine?" Jackie asked. "You can't keep torturing yourself like this?"

"I have nothing else better to do," said Corrine. "What should I be doing, going to lunch with friends and shopping frivolously for shoes?"

"No . . . but you can start baking again. When was the last time you were even at your fondant class?"

"I don't even remember," Corinne admitted.

The next day as Corinne pulled out her mixing bowl and favorite egg beater, she felt as if she'd reconnected with a long-lost friend; the kind of reunion that feels familiar and natural, like no time has passed. The hours slipped by and she lost track of time. Her mind was uncluttered and filled with singular purpose, thinking only about mixing just the right amount of dye into the sugar. Thirteen hours later, Corinne had 150 cake pops. *If I could just turn this into a business . . . make some money . . . be my own boss. . . .*

"Why can't you?" Jackie asked Corinne the next day when Corinne called to tell her friend about her manic episode that had become a saving grace.

"I could never . . . it's just not secure. I'm on my own. I would have to max out credit cards or take out loans or apply for unemployment to get a business started. But really, I'm not *that* good."

So it was with mixed feelings that the weeks passed and Corinne was fueled by her baking. She even did a little networking and found herself designing some new creations for the Communion and Confirmation crowds. Then she received an e-mail from a temp agency. They were sorry they took so long returning her calls, but they found a good temp-to-perm opportunity at an investment firm downtown. Could she be in tomorrow for a trial?

The message was bittersweet. She felt a sudden surge of safety, but that security soon turned to smothering. Could she go for her dream and make her creations cash-worthy? *Should I just do it? I could put up flyers and maybe do a few gratis gigs just to get my name out there.* But her impromptu business plan proved to come too late, as she continued to her next thought: *security is all that counts. . . .*

With a heavy heart, she e-mailed back the temp agency: "I'll be there. What's the address?"

It is certainly understandable that Corinne, a woman on her own with experience in only one domain, would feel uncertain about a career move, especially one involving starting her own business. Corinne lacked the self-esteem to be entrepreneurial, despite her desire to give selling cake pops a go. In her mind it was all or nothing. Either get a job or go for the dream. She chose the job over her own abilities. She allowed her fear and conditioning for security to silence her other ambitions.

If Corinne applied The 5 Living Principles of Well-Being—Commitment, Perseverance, Self-Control, Integrity, and Love—could they have influenced a different outcome for her? Let's see them in action as they apply to building her self-esteem—the kind we all deserve. Let's see how they can help us believe in ourselves so much that we manifest our own safety and destiny, no matter the situation.

Corinne was conflicted because she was fearful. Realizing your destiny comes when you cease to focus on your fear and take responsibility for defining your future. The only thing over which we have control is how we react to circumstances. Had Corinne called upon her Self-Control, she might have been first reminded that her future did not necessarily have to default to "security is everything." Her future is in her hands; she can choose to take charge of herself.

Realizing your destiny comes when you cease to focus on your fear and take responsibility for defining your future.

In considering her situation and relishing in the fact that she actually had some options, Love can be an encouraging compass. I like to say, "Find what you love and a way to make money at it, and you'll never feel like it is work but a calling." Corinne loves to bake and has already found an initial entry point into the business with the Communion and Confirmation customers.

The next step is to make a Commitment. That means creating a business plan and mapping out a reasonable game plan with realistic goals, the steps and timing of its execution, and the means to measure incremental success. A good plan requires monitoring progress through achievement of important milestones. This continuing process is driven by ongoing Perseverance, even when the going gets tough.

To successfully market any product it must be appealing. And a central component of that equation is quality. So, Integrity lends a big hand, creating value in the product as well as attracting, growing, and maintaining a market. No skimping on the ingredients; your customers can always tell.

So for Corinne, the Principles can help her chart a path to finding greater self-worth. And with some additional thought and effort the Principles can be critically relevant as a personal guide to evaluating and making her life decisions as well as providing a template for action. Corinne has within her grasp an ability to martial the power from within herself that is necessary to attain her greater goal of independence and fulfillment.

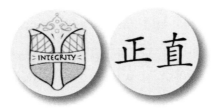

Meet Vicky: Health and Fitness

"Pomp and Circumstance" always made Vicky cry. For some women, the sound of the wedding march might bring a tear, but for Vicky there was always something more moving about the march being played down the graduation aisle than the wedding aisle. Vicky had married young, and while she never regretted her decision to quickly start a family, her opinion was that anyone could get married, but not everyone could graduate. Vicky pondered the meaning of commencement while she waited anxiously to find her daughter in a sea of square black caps, as the graduating class walked double file down the middle of the high school football field. Her daughter was embarking on a new journey in life, just as Vicky was beginning a new phase of her own: empty nesting. Only a short summer stood between Vicky and the day her baby would leave for college—two hours away.

All of Vicky's friends predicted a personal renaissance for her following her daughter's departure. Travel and more disposable income also awaited her, that is if they were right. If their predictions were correct, her love life with her husband, Bob, would also get a jump-start—like they were teenagers again! She chuckled at the thought and then began to believe that perhaps commencement would actually mean that she and Bob did finally take that trip to the Amalfi Coast that they'd talked about back before the kids were born.

Carrying a load of freshly folded whites, she planned her purchase of Rosetta Stone language software to learn Italian as she climbed the staircase of the home she'd made for her family more than twenty-three years ago. The load was a lot lighter now that it was just Bob's and her socks and T-shirts, which didn't explain why she all of a sudden felt light-headed. Petering out at the landing, she leaned against the wall, gasping to catch some air. She was dizzy and sweaty, and her heartbeat was going a little berserk.

Is this a heart attack? A panic attack? Am I really that old?

Dr. Amel looked at Vicky as if he were about to say something he had said a thousand times before.

"Vicky, you are fifty years old, your triglycerides are off the charts, your cholesterol levels are also very high, and I'm worried about your blood pressure. I am prescribing medication for all of it, and I want you to lose at least forty pounds."

Ouch! Vicky didn't know which diagnosis to concern herself with first, but the only thing playing over and over in her head were the words "forty pounds!"

Vicky knew she was overweight, but with three kids and a husband and a house to take care of, she never had time to pay attention to what she ate or to exercise. Back when the house was full and chaotic, most times she wouldn't even sit and eat dinner with the rest of the family; she was too busy setting up and cleaning up to sit down and eat a meal. Late at night when the house fell dark and quiet, Vicky would seek solace in food and television and revel in the little time and privacy she could carve out for herself. Now all she had to show for that comfort was a bad sneak-eating habit and forty pounds to lose, plus a bill of health that was nowhere near clean.

Aside from the reality setting in that her functional age was more like sixty-seven than her biological age of fifty, she felt terrible about how she looked and became lost in a state of self-loathing, which soon led to depression. It had taken years to get here. So she was unmotivated and overwhelmed at the prospect of the effort it would take to undo what time had done. Vicky didn't know where to turn or how to begin getting healthy.

"We can go for walks together or join a gym," Bob suggested.

He was so sweet in wanting to lend his moral and physical support, but really, a gym? Vicky hated the dull idea of organized exercise. To her it meant deliberately spending forty-five minutes a day working out, and she felt further humiliated by her shape and "oversized" body. Besides, she was always hungry, so a diet wouldn't work. It was far too limiting. There was no hope. In fact, when it came to finding a fit and healthful lifestyle, she was already defeated. Vicky believed she had no choices and no chance to change her ways, and in her pursuit to avoid the truth, she hid behind a wall of excuses.

Bob was floored by Vicky's lack of will and ambition, and they fought about how worried he was for her health. Vicky's mind was made up: it was simply too late. Her prime had passed anyway. What was she going to do? Lose forty pounds and run a marathon? *Please.*

Vicky, the self-proclaimed "middle-aged fat lady," filed the trip to the Amalfi Coast under "D" for "Dream," as she retreated into a sea of withdrawal and bitter acceptance that kept her as far away from health and happiness as she was from the Mediterranean.

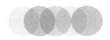

In the face of the unknown Vicky crumbled. Her doctor wanted her to move out of her comfort zone in order to establish a healthier lifestyle. Overwhelmed by the reality of how unhealthy she was, Vicky swept the seriousness under the rug and allowed excuse-making and denial to take over. The 5 Living Principles of Well-Being are a fantastic tool to utilize, especially when fear and doubt threaten to overwhelm and take over. By implementing The 5 Living Principles, Vicky could have found the courage to take baby steps.

It seems that Vicky's biggest challenge was not the weight but the denial. As a devoted wife and mother, she had created a certain routine and was lulled into a pattern that justified a certain lack of personal attention with which she also became comfortable. When all of your efforts are focused on the care of others, it is easy to lose sight of how important it is to care for yourself. You might even be aware of the situation but feel it is just too difficult to do anything about it.

Perhaps while she was making good choices for everyone else, Vicky, too, sensed she was not doing the same for herself. Maintaining a healthy lifestyle takes a bit of planning and discipline. Maybe she allowed herself to slip or become somewhat complacent where her own well-being was concerned because it was just an easier justifiable choice.

When all of your efforts are focused on the care of others, it is easy to lose sight of how important it is to care for yourself.

To turn her around and jump-start a new reality, Vicky will need to call on her Integrity. She has to stop and be honest with herself about how she got to where she is. Sure, caring for her family took time and effort, but no one would have faulted her for taking the time to care for herself. She also cannot really claim ignorance. She has always valued education, but it would seem that she has not made smart decisions. She also might have gotten a bit lazy, and that includes her diet. Vicky needs to quickly admit these things to herself before anything else. Her self-denial must give way to self-analysis and coming to grips with the real reasons for her present condition.

Self-evaluation opens the door to Self-Control and taking responsibility for the choices you have made and their consequences. Vicky must accept that she allowed herself, even gave herself permission, to gain forty pounds. It was the lifestyle she alone chose. However, the Breakthrough is that it is a lifestyle she can alter. Her daughter's departure is a real opportunity to set better goals—a healthy new beginning awaits.

Bob's suggestions come from a place of Love. However, her fighting him does not reflect her love for him, nor does her conduct set a good example for anyone. She also has to learn to forgive herself for the past, open her heart, and care enough about her own health and well-being. Vicky must realize she has to be good to herself in order to be good for others. And given her doctor's concerns, it is better for her to begin late than never at all.

In Vicky's case, the early stages of applying the Principles really deal with mental and emotional assessment and realization. The next phase is action. Her Commitment is required to adopt a practical plan that addresses attainable goals for her through proper diet, nutrition, and exercise. A smart move would be for Vicky to announce her intentions to select friends and family and work with professionals to help chart her course. Admitting it to others makes the Commitment real. Vicky might also be surprised to find how proud of herself she might feel for wanting to do something like this and how proud and supportive of her others will be when she tells them.

To make her transformation successful, Vicky must have Perseverance. It keeps her on the right path when self-doubt and difficulty arise—and they will. It is a natural part of the journey. Vicky must face it with determination . . . no way out but through. . . . The people with whom she shares her Commitment now also become cheerleaders—motivating and rewarding her ongoing efforts with positive energy. It is the perfect fuel for Vicky's health-filled new direction.

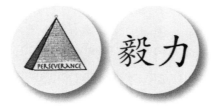

Meet Regina: Work-Life Balance

Regina tossed from her right side to her left, punched the pillow in frustration, and stared at the clock beside her bed. It was 2:45 AM, and the house was quiet as a mouse, with the exception of the thoughts that raced through her head. She couldn't shut them off, and they were made more annoying by the sleeping sounds and slight snores coming from her husband, Bart, who lay beside her. This is the way it went for Regina night after night.

In fact, Regina hadn't had a good night's sleep since the third trimester of her first pregnancy, just a little more than two years ago. She had held out hope she'd sleep a full night as soon as she stopped nursing her second baby, who just turned seven months; but that was already three months ago, and still she had a nightly date with her clock.

After Regina went back to work teaching ninth grade at the school where she'd worked for eight years, she began to experience panic attacks. At first she thought her heart palpitations were from all of the coffee she was consuming: Getting up at 5:00 AM to get the kids off to her mother's for the day, after only finally falling asleep at 3:30ish, Regina inhaled coffee to keep herself from falling asleep at her desk. By 3:00 PM she'd have downed five cups, which she realized not only caused her heart to race and her head to pound, but kept her from normal sleep-wake cycles.

But despite her addiction to coffee, the doctor diagnosed Regina with panic attacks and prescribed her Paxil to "even her out." And she noticed the attacks were worse when she left the babies for the day. She experienced a desperate inner struggle between her maternal side and her ambitious side, and beat herself up for having to work. As the bills piled up, Regina and Bart made the decision for them both to take side jobs. She, as a tutor, and he, as a house painter on the weekends once the weather warmed up.

When her girlfriends called her, she was either in class or at a student's house for tutoring. She couldn't call them back because by the time she got home, she wanted to see her children, feed them, bathe them, and read them some stories before she tucked one child in and rocked the other. She and Bart didn't eat dinner until 9:00 every night, so they could have some intimate conversation. And when it came to the physical side of their love life, Regina had given up. She was too wound up and distracted to even think about being close with her husband. By the time the 11:00 news came on, she knew she wouldn't be reaching out to any girlfriends that day, and she felt isolated and alone. *How can I be in such a loving marriage and be blessed with two beautiful boys and feel so lonely?* she wondered.

Talking to or seeing her girlfriends weren't the only things Regina missed. She missed her runs. They weren't too long, but always three or four times a week. She'd alternate between 5Ks (3.2 miles) and 6-milers, and on the weekends she would run some local charitable races. But that was before her last pregnancy, and now she yearned for the endorphins that used to give her a rush.

No friends, no exercise, just round-the-clock overdrive. Regina felt depleted.

"You must make time for yourself, Regina," her therapist, Carol, told her. "If you don't, you won't be good for your husband or your babies."

"It's not so easy," Regina cried. "I have two kids and two jobs, and my marriage is important to me, so I'd rather spend time cultivating that when I have any spare time than getting my nails done."

"If you can find time to come here, Regina, then you can get creative and figure out a way to get a run in or go to lunch with a friend. You have absolutely no balance in your life. You're going to crash, if you don't find some soon, and then where will that leave you? Where will it leave your family, when you can't function for them?"

"Is my time up, yet?" Regina asked impatiently.

"Only if you want it to be."

"Yes, I want it to be. I need to go grocery shopping before I take the kids to their music class."

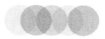

Regina's therapist gave her good advice, but unfortunately Regina wasn't about to take it. She had become so accustomed to caring for others, especially her family, that she was neglecting the most important person of all. She simply couldn't see the way through her hectic life. Regina's work-life struggle is a pervasive one amongst many women, and The 5 Living Principles of Well-Being could be a helpful tool to guide Regina to a more centered life. Let's see how.

In some situations of difficulty, certain individual Principles may be more immediately relevant than others. Nonetheless, each in its turn at some future point may still become important to complete the solution. In classic fashion, Regina faces the work-life balancing act, complete with all the frustrations and self-guilt that come with it. Left unaddressed, Regina's therapist is right. She is on her way to "crashing."

This common dilemma is encouraged by what we women have come to feel is our job—our responsibility to do everything and for everyone. It is not just about ambition, but the notion has grown that we can and must "do it all," and I want to say that is just not a realistic or healthy way to live. You create a constant state of stress for yourself. No wonder Regina can't sleep; she can't turn it off.

Much of how we live life is about the choices we make. If you find yourself saying, "I want it all, but I can't do it all," then perhaps you shouldn't. To do otherwise can lead to insurmountable obstacles to physical and mental well-being.

Coffee alone is not the culprit, and no wonder she struggles to be intimate with her husband. Regina can't live with the stress she has put on herself. So she needs to give it a break.

Her ambitions for work, family, and personal time are admirable but not entirely realistic. First, she must tune her emotions to a different frequency and Love herself. She also needs to accept she cannot do everything she wants to do. Regina's attempt to be Superwoman is of her own creation, albeit perhaps further encouraged by today's cultural pressures. However, she must ignore the peer pressure and focus on forgiving herself if she is unable to completely fulfill the role of superhuman.

With some renewed Self-Control . . . prioritize what is truly most important.

Regina has been caught up in the race rather than

taking charge of it and dictating the pace. With some renewed Self-Control she can prioritize what is truly most important to her. In her case, it sounds like money is tight and both spouses need two jobs to make ends meet. If that is the case and the budget is already as lean as it can be, then Regina must accept that. It does not mean she loves her family any less or is any less of a woman or a success. And visits with the girls might have to take a backseat for now over something like fitting in some regular exercise for herself instead. Maybe she can meet the girls at a health club periodically for a workout together and kill two birds with one stone—it just takes a bit of planning.

Regina's situation is about understanding, forgiveness, and accepting herself, which are all attributes of Love and Self-Control. It is good to aim high, but continue to be reasonable. She has the tools to take charge of her destiny and define it by terms that make it work for her. Regina's life, like all of ours, is fluid, and so must be her priorities and plans.

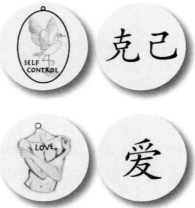

Meet Denise: Aging

Denise fastened the buttons of her black man-tailored blouse from bottom to top while staring at her hands in the full-length mirror. As her fingers twisted their way upward, she couldn't help but be horrified by the new veins that were popping from her bony hands. Her hands resembled her mother's, which reminded Denise not only of how she was getting on in years, but of how much she missed her mom who had passed almost two years ago.

Getting older was always something that Denise grappled with. She was never a fan of birthdays, hers or anyone else's, and strongly disagreed with the philosophy "age is just a number." Next month her number would be forty-eight, and with her mother gone now and nobody to take care of, she felt hollow and confused about her place in the world and what happens next.

"So, what do you want to do for your birthday?" Marie asked Denise while dipping her fork into a side of balsamic vinaigrette before piercing it into her salad.

"You've known me since we're eleven, Marie, why would you even bother to ask me that?"

"I just never understood what your issue is with birthdays."

"I don't want to get old," Denise admitted flatly. "And now I'm actually starting to look like I'm about to hit the wall. Fifty is just staring me in the face, and you want me to somehow feel good about it."

"Well, gee, if you put it that way, D . . . you really need a reality check."

"The reality is, Marie, I walk into a room and feel invisible to men . . . heck, even to women. I hear the word ma'am now everywhere I go, and I feel like my boobs might as well be sitting on my knees, except now my knees are acting up, so they probably couldn't handle the extra weight! I can't read the cell phone bill, even when I squint. And when I squint, my face looks like a landing pad for crows. Whoever said, 'Getting old ain't for sissies,' sure was right. I'm more than halfway to the grave now. And that scares the life out of me!"

"Denise, you can't obsess about dying," Marie scolded. "You can't waste away your life in fear of when your life will end. For that matter, you might as well already be dead. What a terrible paradox to have created for yourself, Denise. You're missing the bigger picture—wasting the journey."

Getting defensive, Denise said, "I don't want to hear it. I don't want to celebrate my birthday, and I don't want to talk about this anymore."

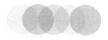

What is the bigger picture? Can The 5 Living Principles of Well-Being help Denise see it, while transforming her view on aging and overcoming her fear of the physical and emotional changes she is experiencing?

Denise clearly sees herself as a victim of time. We all easily see that. Even her friend rightly encourages Denise to focus on the journey, not the destination, but Denise can't or won't try to see it. Her negativity is further reinforced by the natural effects of aging we all experience.

Denise needs to change the tape in her head. No one likes getting older. But we can still find value, beauty, and joy in all it has to offer if we approach this inevitable process with Love. The grace and dignity Denise will require to help her cope and find a positive direction only flow from an open mind and heart. Right now Denise is simply being closed-minded. She needs to refocus her attention from worrying about her future to loving herself enough to take good care of herself. Only then can she begin to engage in the more positive thoughts and behavior that will improve her overall wellness. A shift in attitude is not always instant pudding. Denise may also need the support and encouragement of friends, but the transformation can begin when Denise opens up to the possibility her future holds.

Denise also seems to be in a bit of a panic mode. A little Self-Control might help with her composure. However, she still must come to accept the fact that while we all feel empathy for her on this subject, not everyone reacts the same way she does. Denise has options, things she can do to improve her physical and mental condition and enhance the quality of her life. She cannot defeat time, and in trying to do so she will only defeat herself. There are certain things we can control and others we simply cannot, and aging is most obviously one of those matters that is out of our hands.

Notwithstanding, Denise needs to take responsibility for what she *can* do to help herself. It sounds like the first option might be for her to plan some regular exercise and maybe even get some contact lenses for her blurred vision. These efforts can go a long way in raising her self-esteem and providing, quite literally, a better outlook on life.

Denise feels coming up on age fifty is a big crossroads for her. Some of us may put that number a little higher or lower but we understand how she feels. I have met people who at thirty-five seem older and others at sixty who are younger. It's a number. Thinking young helps you to stay young. It's mind over matter, and there are countless examples of people who have staved off disease or still accomplish

I have met people who at thirty-five seem older and others at sixty who are younger. It's a number. Thinking young helps you to stay young.

mental and physical feats that might otherwise be daunting to their younger counterparts.

Thinking young is getting up and doing things—both things you like and those you don't like to do. It is not giving in—not stopping, keeping busy, not vegging out but being productive. Grab life for all it's worth, with its ups and downs, and know you are not alone. If you are really living and not just sitting on the sidelines, this is what life is all about.

Moving along with life takes Commitment—regardless of the circumstances—to live life the best we can. That means we are dedicated to staying in the game, and whether it is Denise or any of us, some days will not be the greatest; we know that is just the way it is. So at times it might take a little more Perseverance, but every effort should reflect Integrity. In all we do, we get out what we put in. Denise must make the promise to herself to embrace the race and remain true to her course.

Aging and how we handle it is a particularly sensitive subject. Clearly it is not to be taken lightly, nor can we oversimplify the response to someone's feelings about it. There are whole books devoted to the subject. But in order for us to maximize the experience of living, most of these books will likely conclude with the simple truth that only action can replace fear. Denise is clearly stuck in a rut and believes she is powerless to do anything about it. If she can just take the Principles to heart and begin to apply them, they can help nudge her out of her funk and forward on the right road to fulfillment.

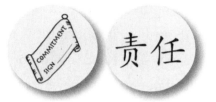

Embrace It, Own It, Live It®

We cannot do anything about the past. We need to forgive ourselves and not be fearful that we do not immediately have all the answers. However, the opportunities and answers you seek in life are there waiting for you. For the four women above, the process of self-discovery was very personal. The road traveled is different for each of us. In this book, I have shared my journey and the powerful ally I have found that works for me and the others who have embraced it.

But what I will also share with you is there is nothing new under the sun, and each of us must find the tools that are right for us to realize the fundamental idea of who we want to be. There is no secret formula, instant pudding, or magic wand that leads you to your Breakthrough.

Finding empowerment, fulfillment, and well-being takes self-reflection, desire, and a willingness to grow. The great thing is that as you embrace The 5 Living Principles of Well-Being and SheaNetics, both will be there for you every step of the way.

I can talk to you about how important it is to learn to be in the moment if you are going to experience mind-body transformations— to be able to shift your thoughts to somewhere within yourself where you can analyze, evaluate, discover, and break through. I can tell you how The 5 Living Principles of Well-Being can facilitate and empower this process as well as add value to whatever else you do in life. However, just as these Principles reside in all of us, only you can tap into them and make them work for you. How do you do that? Where do you begin? You must *Embrace It, Own It, Live It*®.

Shea Vaughn's Breakthrough! is really about The 5 Living Principles of Well-Being, the mental philosophy behind SheaNetics, and how it combines with its unique physical routines to create a healthy lifestyle that promotes a state of well-being just for you. We call them "Living" Principles because they are alive. They are a positive part of us all and with each of us wherever we are.

We say SheaNetics is "Your Pathway to Well-Being." It is a best friend. But your personal journey to that destination can only begin when you *Embrace It*. Be open, wrap your arms around SheaNetics, its principles, and the healthy lifestyle it represents with the same spirit of Commitment you would give to anything you value and hold dear. Bring it close to you, into your heart, and hug it like you would a cherished child. *Own It* by showing Self-Control and accepting your responsibility to do what is good for you and have the Perseverance and Integrity to do it the best you are able. *Live It.* Set a good example and reveal the quality person you are by using SheaNetics as your guide to everyday life. It's made great changes in my life and I promise it will in yours.

> *"Embrace It,*
>
> *Own It,*
>
> *Live It®"*

For example, let me share an experience I had with my son Vince when I decided to really *live* life. The United States Army Parachute Team, commonly referred to as the "Golden Knights," was officially established in 1961, two years following its earlier formation at Fort Bragg, North Carolina, for the purpose of competing in a skydiving competition that was dominated by international talent. The team grew from thirteen to ninety members and is comprised of pilots and support personnel that make about 100 appearances a year.

One of the Golden Knights events was at the Chicago Air & Water Show, the largest spectator event in the United States and the largest ongoing show of its kind in North America. Each summer for one week in August, more than two million people flock to the shores of Lake Michigan for the event.

My son Vince accepted an invitation to do a tandem jump out of an airplane with the Golden Knights. The jump was to take place on Saturday, August 14, 2010. I was at Vince's house the evening before. We were chatting about the jump when he looked up at me and said, "Hey, Mom, why don't you jump with me?"

I looked at him, paused for a second, and said, "Wow, that would be great!"

We were both excited about doing it together. Driving home I remember thinking this certainly wasn't something I had on my bucket list, but what a great opportunity to jump out of an airplane, and to do it with my son. I really didn't have much time to think about it, because we were being picked up at his place at 7:30 the next morning. So when I got home I shared it with my husband, Steve, who was somewhat surprised, but then said, "Go for it!"

We were picked up early the next morning and taken to the Gary Jet Center of the Gary-Chicago Airport in Gary, Indiana, where we began our orientation. Vince and I were seated at a table and introduced to the Golden Knights team. Each team member stepped forward individually, stating his name and the personal story that led him to join the U.S. Army and further pursue the opportunity to become a Golden Knight. It was impressive and heartwarming to hear the details of their journeys, but even more evident was the unmistakable love and protection they all felt for one another. Constantly, they slapped each other on the back, gave high-fives, fist bumps, and encouragement like, "Everything is great," "Ready to go," and "Nice job." They included Vince and me in all of it.

According to the team, each member stands for Loyalty—Duty—Respect—Selfless Service—Honor—Integrity—Personal Courage. They certainly exemplified these words and believed it was not only their duty but their honor to defend their homeland, the United States of America, against all odds and for all the right reasons, and to preserve our rights and way of life. All of it impressed me and certainly added to our comfort level. *If you're going to jump out of a plane*, I kept thinking, *it just doesn't get any better than this.*

It was time to get ready to climb aboard a Fokker C-31A Friendship for our jump. So before taking our places on the plane they brought us some unattractive bright yellow jumpsuits to put on and then snapped and tied us all together. Vince and I were pretty relaxed and taking it all in. Vince was doing his jump with Staff Sergeant Joe Abein, and I was with Team Leader Michael Elliott, Sergeant First Class . . . two outstanding men.

We boarded the aircraft with excitement and continued to enjoy the positive chat and great attitudes the team exuded. I was sitting next to Vince when he turned to me and said, "Mom, don't be nervous, because this will be over so fast, and you don't want to waste your time on being nervous. Just enjoy the time we have together, just you and me."

> "Mom, don't be nervous, because this will be over so fast, and you don't want to waste your time on being nervous. Just enjoy the time we have together, just you and me."

How right he was. It was the most amazing time together 13,000 feet in the air, ready to jump out and experience the wind in your face, the freedom of space. I was creating a memory with my son that I would hold in my heart forever.

Michael and I got up and approached the door hooked together. I stood at the open doorway as we got our final staging commands before leaping from the plane, ". . . READY. SET. GO . . . !"

Out we jumped.

As we were falling, Joe and Vince took their jump out of the plane, and soon they were right across from us. We were waving and putting our thumbs up to indicate all was wonderful. We got so close together we could look straight into each other's eyes and share the exhilaration of the moment. Down we floated and landed on the beach just north of Oak Street Beach. Vince and I both had big smiles on our faces, and we hugged each

Vince and I both had big smiles on our faces, and we hugged each other, acknowledging without words that we were grateful for this once-in-a-lifetime moment together.

other, acknowledging without words that we were grateful for this once-in-a-lifetime moment together. I felt love beyond words and gave thanks to my son for the invitation to be part of this cherished flight.

Jumping out of a plane took courage and trust, as well as a desire to take risks and experience things that are out of my comfort zone. I may have jumped out of a plane, something that I really never considered doing before, but I find this experience a useful metaphor for how SheaNetics and The 5 Living Principles of Well-Being enhance my life: I took the proverbial plunge into the vastness of life's unknown, let the wind hit me square in the face, and relished in it. Do not be afraid of the freefall, and take note that the landing never kills you. In the end, the ground is soft, the grass is sweet, and the lessons learned are worth applying to future endeavors that you are now equipped to take.

CHAPTER SEVEN

Connecting the Dots: the Anatomy, the Principles, and Well-Being

*If you always put limit[s] on everything
you do, physical or anything else, it will spread into
your work and into your life. There are no limits.
There are only plateaus, and you must not stay
there, you must go beyond them.*

—Bruce Lee

In the last chapter we examined the challenges facing four individuals, a very different and personal issue for each person. We left them experiencing their Breakthroughs using The 5 Living Principles of Well-Being. We saw how the Principles, when engaged, could guide them in each of their situations to clearer reasoning, a more informed perspective, and a positive direction. As a result, they could face their truths and find hope for their futures.

You know from all I have shared with you how to recognize, be open, and find truth through experiencing Breakthroughs and why the Anatomy is so essential to leading you to your Breakthrough. However, it is the Principles that call you to action and motivate you to adopt healthy lifestyle changes that will become everlasting. It is the Principles that are at the center of all your efforts and choices. Now you have the tools and the desire to put them to good use—to find wellness and create well-being in your life.

Early in the book I said the Anatomy of a Breakthrough is a method of instruction, an outline that helps you to recall and think through the things that matter to you. It shows you how to be in the moment and seek out Breakthroughs. It is important because it helps you to tune out your many distractions and begin to focus on what is important if you want to create and maintain personal wellness in your life. It is a meditative process you can use to simply give stress a break and bring on a little peacefulness or apply it to resolving more serious issues that profoundly affect you.

Applying the Anatomy and The 5 Living Principles

The Anatomy is there to help you focus and think objectively, but the real drivers of positive action and personal enrichment are The 5 Living Principles of Well-Being. I envision an ever-present "heart of enlightenment" emitting five separate streams of brightly lit beads, each representing one of the Principles, that shine down continuously upon you to inspire, motivate, and direct all of your actions. The Principles encourage you to be open to Breakthroughs, and they enrich your cognitive thinking and the process we call the Anatomy of a Breakthrough.

The Principles are there to guide you through all you think, feel, and encounter in life, giving structure and meaning to all you do. This is powerful. Many people seek order, reason, and purpose, which are what The 5 Living Principles help you to achieve. This provides balance and wellness, which are essential to creating a state of well-being in your life.

The Principles are there to guide you through all you think, feel, and encounter in life, giving structure and meaning to all you do.

Scott's Story

In a recent SheaNetics class, Scott, who was one of my regular students, shared his experience of how The 5 Living Principles of Well-Being helped him through a challenging time and a tough decision. In his story, you will see that his Breakthrough was the very application of the Principles; equally important, his experience also illustrates how the Anatomy helped him to divert his attention from the negativity and distraction of the situation in which he found himself, to redirect his concentration, and shift his perception. The Anatomy and the Principles helped him to forge ahead with grace, dignity, self-esteem, and a renewed hope for his future. Here is Scott's account:

● ● ●

A week ago I was laid off from my job. In fact, Friday was my last day, and before I got the bad news, I had been spearheading a project that was not yet completed. Once the message had been delivered, I sat at my desk struggling with the decision whether to finish it or leave it for someone else to do. I had trepidation about walking away from something I (had) started.

I also felt uneasy about the uncertainty Monday would bring, as I would begin the next workweek without work, and I thought about how easy it would be—even expected—to just stick it to them, leaving the work undone. But what quickly came to mind was Shea's voice talking about The 5 Living Principles of Well-Being, as she does in each SheaNetics class I take. After considering the meaning of each one of them—Commitment, Perseverance, Self-Control, Integrity, and Love—I decided to stay and finish the project before leaving.

I chose to keep my Commitment to show up and do the right thing. I was still being compensated for the day's work, so I found the Perseverance and Self-Control to complete the project. I overcame what could have been a day of defeat and took responsibility to carry on as I felt any real professional would. I felt that I was being true to my honest nature and good name by following through with quality work, which helped me live the Principle of Integrity.

When I left that day and said good-bye to my office mates, I actually felt at peace; I knew I (had) made the right choice and set the best example, and I Loved myself for that. I applied all 5 Living Principles and left the office empowered, centered, focused, and ready to address other challenges in my life—

known and unknown—with a healthier and more positive atti-tude and perspective.

• • •

We all sat quietly in class, admiring Scott's honesty, and we were grateful to him for sharing his story. Ann, another student, turned to Scott, her eyes welled up with tears, and she said, "Thank you, Scott. I frequently feel overwhelmed with my daily responsibilities of family and work, but your story reinforces for me that the Principles are here to help guide me through all my stressful moments."

Well said, Ann. The 5 Living Principles of Well-Being are a catalyst to set you on the right path, and they are what keep you there. What Scott did in the face of a career challenge was to use the Principles to help him choose a response that would provide him with an enriching experience instead of keeping him prisoner to negative patterns and self-destruc-tive thoughts.

Listening to Scott's story, we might feel as though the Anatomy played a lesser role, but it was still very much at work. Scott shared with us that his first reaction to what happened to him was totally emotional; however, he knew this response was unproductive. Steadying himself, he shifted his thoughts to the moment and started to analyze the situation. The Anatomy helped him to focus and come to a realization, which allowed him to invite a Breakthrough.

Nevertheless, it was the Principles that inspired action and gave deeper meaning to his experience. The SheaNetics 5 Living Principles of Well-Being help you to find your center and the wherewithal to accomplish the duties and tasks that lay before you. You can do this without fear and indecision because your open heart is the inspiration for your decisions and actions.

Scott had a Breakthrough because he called upon The Principles to guide his decision and direct his actions. His Breakthrough was doing the right thing, and it helped him because he loved himself more. Breakthroughs drive results. Scott acted in accordance with his true honest nature and was rewarded with a sense of inner peace, self-worth, and acceptance, putting him one step closer to achieving a personal state of well-being.

Vicky's Story

Let's take another look at Vicky from Chapter 6. You will recall that her daughter was graduating and that Vicky was making plans for a fantasy trip to the Amalfi Coast with her lovable husband, Bob. However, she came face-to-face with some health issues that just might derail the dream from becoming reality.

The situation Vicky found herself in is, unfortunately, much too common. Throughout the years of caring for her family, Vicky had gained forty pounds, and the extra weight was now posing a real threat to both her physical and mental well-being. Her husband, along with her doctor, was trying in a caring way to make her conscious of the issue. Yet even though she met their efforts with apparent resistance, it's hard to believe that in all those years of making good choices for everyone else, Vicky did not sense the need to do the same for herself.

When Vicky felt out of breath simply from carrying a little laundry up some steps, it was a wake-up call that she began to answer. It made her stop and shift her focus from housework to her health, using the Anatomy to become aware of what was at stake. Vicky began to ask herself, "Is this going to be my destiny? Am I prediabetic, as the doctor says, and what quality of life can I look forward to?" She began to realize that in the process of taking care of everyone else's needs, she had neglected her own.

Vicky began to acknowledge that she could have benefited much sooner if she had understood the importance of making time for herself along the way. She could also see how she might have altogether avoided the issues she now faced. Notably, too, Vicky came to admit to herself that her choices had not all been unconscious ones. This was partly just an excuse for not making the effort. She was now at the point of revelation and on the verge of a Breakthrough. The Anatomy had invited her to have this experience, but as you read in Chapter 6, it was the Principles that would make it happen and that are the drivers of lasting change.

Vicky owes her Breakthrough to the Integrity and Self-Control she exhibited when she was honest with herself about the circumstances leading to her weight gain and when she accepted the responsibility for it. Her plan to lose weight and get healthy would require fervent Commitment and Perseverance when her fortitude weakened. Along the way, however, her efforts would be constantly bolstered by Love as well as her desire to be better and to set the best example she could for her family and her friends.

Bring It with You:
Make Time for Yourself

What if I told you that the activities you loved to do in your youth could be valuable to you right now? Things like dancing, painting, swimming, playing a musical instrument, or any other fun-loving activity that kept you thinking and moving back then can motivate you now. Of course, you may not be able to do the activity with the same speed or agility, but that is to be expected. The point is that you can "bring it with you"—that is, you can feel and regain some of the physical and mental joy and benefit you previously experienced in your youth.

Although many people—especially women—forgo these passions and feel guilty or selfish for taking time for themselves, the truth is that making time for activities like these boosts your brain, lowers your stress level, and enriches your life. How many times have you heard someone say, "I wish I'd kept up my piano lessons"? Some may regret having lacked the foresight or the means to continue, or they may have parents they blame for making the decision for them. Whatever the situation, at this point it is all in the past, and the important issue is what you can do about it now. You can "bring it with you." It's never too late.

We all have regrets, but with the right inspiration we have the opportunity to turn those negative feelings into something positive. The 5 Living Principles of Well-Being do just that. Commitment, Perseverance, Self-Control, Integrity, and Love are all you need to put a plan together and "bring it with you." Each Principle guides you through this fulfilling undertaking. What do you have to lose? Whatever you accomplish will certainly be more than if you had put forth no effort. Do something you never thought you would. Rediscover something you miss. It can give you a great sense of pride and satisfaction. What a boost to your well-being!

We all have regrets, but with the right inspiration we have the opportunity to turn those negative feelings into something positive.

The activities may differ, but the concept is the same. Students come up to me all the time and say, "Wow, what fun! I haven't done a roll or a head-stand since college." At whatever point you realize you wish you could do

171

something you used to enjoy, "bring it with you" is the key to taking the first step in making this happen. What you thought was lost can now be found. Apply the Principles and watch what wonderful physical and mental benefits you can experience.

Your Pathway to Well-Being

A healthy mind, body, and heart are the components of wellness. You create well-being by connecting these elements, just as the sounds of individual musicians playing in an orchestra are blended into one glorious symphony by the conductor. The various stages of the Anatomy of a Breakthrough are the instruments through which the music of your mind, body, and heart can speak. You are the orchestra of musicians, and The 5 Living Principles of Well-Being are your conductor. The harmoniously pleasing symphony of sound that is created is a metaphor for the sense of well-being that can be yours when you embrace the SheaNetics lifestyle.

An instrument is nothing without a musician to give it life, and to make music that is transcendent and moves you to a better place takes diligent effort and training that is inspirational. As you use the Anatomy and allow the Principles to be ever present in your life and to guide your mind, body, and heart, Breakthroughs occur organically, and you begin to make better decisions overall. This leads to experiencing positive, mind-body transformations that form the foundation for a lasting lifestyle of wellness.

SheaNetics is your pathway to well-being. It is a mind-body lifestyle practice. We have thoroughly explored the mental and emotional aspects, but as Vicky found out, you can achieve balance and well-being only when you make a similar effort to improve the overall health of your body.

SheaNetics posits that a healthy body is created not by exercise alone but by the *right approach* to exercise. Adding cardio exercise (such as walking, running, cycling, jumping rope, or swimming) at least twice a week is definitely important for the proper functioning of your heart, lungs, and metabolism. However, the goal is to exercise the whole body. So how do you maximize the benefits of your efforts? SheaNetics is the perfect complement to any other form of exercise or physical practice.

The Importance of Whole-Body Exercise

In order to achieve mind-body wellness, you need to exercise the whole body and the mind. The choreography of all SheaNetics workouts takes advantage of my multidisciplinary fitness background to compose a physical mix that is always fresh and produces a full-body experience with real results.

Everyone wants strong core muscles. SheaNetics introduces you to the body-enhancing benefits of Tri-Core Power Training, a highly effective technique for developing all three regions of the core to improve balance and boost physical performance. Tri-Core Power Training builds up and tones the three core regions of the body: the abdominal muscles and pelvic and lower back areas that help support the spine. It is beneficial for everyone because it helps to improve or maintain mobility and balance and can prevent injuries. It is valuable to any person at any level of training and physical activity, particularly to performance-driven athletes who have to excel to stay in the game.

Maintaining a strong core is critical to all of us as we age. A good core encourages correct posture and improves stability when sitting, standing, and walking, which greatly influences the quality of life by improving one's range of motion and helping to prevent falls and other similar accidents and injuries. Some of my students who suffer from lower back problems have reported that SheaNetics has helped decrease soreness and, in many cases, eliminated it altogether.

SheaNetics Signature:
Why Stretching Is So Important

Stretching enhances the quality, effectiveness, and safety of all physical activity and should be incorporated naturally as a general practice into the design of any workout. Yet most individuals and even athletes unfortunately make the same common mistake: they pursue fitness by concentrating on aerobic and weight-training activities that compress and shorten muscles without incorporating stretching or not stretching enough. These enthusiasts consider stretching inconvenient, or they are simply unaware of the substantial fitness gains to be made by stretching. Too few seem to understand that stretching is as essential as aerobic and weight-training activities. Stretching returns muscles to their original length and can even further lengthen, strengthen, and condition the muscles beyond their original state if the individual increases the amount and degree of the stretch as well as the length of time the move is held. Most important, stretching enhances range of motion, helps to prevent injury, and improves injury recovery.

A typical workout has three phases: the warm-up, the workout activity, and the cool-down. Stretching should be added to the first and last phases. The primary purpose of the warm-up is to prepare the body and the mind for more strenuous activity. You should take five to ten minutes to warm up, but remember that this is not an exact science, so it may vary a bit by individual. Begin by stretching your legs, back, shoulders, neck, and arms. If you are going for a jog, you will want to do some light walking. This increases your heart rate and the body's core and muscle temperatures, and it prepares you for more vigorous exercise.

At the end of your jog or other workout activity, you enter the cool-down, in which you stretch again. This phase is important because it not only brings your blood into areas to help with the removal of lactic acid, it also helps to safely lower your heart rate to a resting pulse. Again, five to ten minutes is recommended, starting with slowing down to a comfortable walk if you are jogging, and then stretching.

Most important, stretching enhances range of motion, helps to prevent injury, and improves injury recovery.

In SheaNetics, we know the valuable effect a good stretch can have on both the mind and the body. It is one of the cornerstones of SheaNetics and is seamlessly integrated into its poses and free-flowing sequences. In addition to building flexibility, SheaNetics embraces muscle endurance and strength training while inspiring you to focus and improve mental awareness, thereby achieving most of your fitness goals with a full-body workout in a reasonably short amount of time.

There are three basic types of stretches and you will find all three in my SheaNetics workouts:

- **Static.** The most common stretch, a static stretch, calls for simply placing the body in the required position and holding the stretch for ten to thirty seconds. This is safe and effective because there is no further movement or bouncing once the position is established.

- **Passive.** Range of motion is increased through the use of external force during a passive stretch. The body begins a stretch normally but is further encouraged into a deeper execution through the introduction of a partner, a wall, the floor, or another prop.

- **Dynamic.** The dynamic stretch uses momentum, such as a leg swing. Ballistic stretches are also included in this category. These movements are most relevant to sports-related activities such as gymnastics[1] or martial arts.

Each SheaNetics workout is built on individual positions, or poses, joined into movements that are coupled into sequences. Each sequence is then linked in a compatible and seamless fashion. The SheaNetics student finds that a given series of movements, once perceived as separate, fully engages one's attention, and the class feels like one continuous flowing movement.

Meanwhile, on a subliminal level, when you move a muscle, it creates a memory of that activity. This is known as *muscle memory*. So even as the order of movements and the sequences of each workout

---

[1] Stretching Types and Stages, http://www.momentumsports.co.uk/TtStretching1.asp

change, the muscle's memory retention helps the body to recognize each move. Whenever the body next encounters the move, it reacts positively to the stimulation and moves more efficiently, thus allowing you to further challenge yourself by raising the quality of the movement's execution.

This muscle awareness is the key to advancing the physical benefits of SheaNetics training. The body is now relaxed, energized, and open to optimizing the execution of the sequence, and with more effort comes better results. SheaNetics works the entire body, and you'll feel as though you have just given yourself an energizing massage. What a gift!

SheaNetics is also effective in improving your mental and emotional condition. This lies in a subtle truth we discussed earlier, which is well documented by Eastern practices and Western scientific studies. We know that meditation reduces stress, promoting many physical and mental benefits like relaxation, calm, and peace[2]—a sense of well-being. A SheaNetics workout is so different from anything you are used to doing. It immediately centers your thoughts and efforts on the execution of its flowing sequences. This demands your complete attention and commitment, and the great thing is that you can do it. Through its ability to positively focus the mind and body in this way,

---

[2] Ibid.

SheaNetics is *meditation in motion and thought*—lengthening muscles, strengthening the body, reducing stress, and further encouraging you along "Your Pathway to Well-Being."

SheaNetics exercise can make a substantial contribution to your wellness when you make it a normal part of a healthy lifestyle. The 5 Living Principles of Well-Being are also a big part of the SheaNetics exercise routines; they motivate and challenge you to do your best, and they add meaning to what you are doing and what you want to achieve. Most important, the Principles help you to think that a daily Commitment to your physical fitness, while crucial to your health, is just a natural part of the process of living. When it is part of your lifestyle, it doesn't feel like effort. It simply feels great.

The 5 Living Principles of Well-Being are a big impetus to creating a healthy lifestyle for yourself—naturally. The first step is making a Commitment to exercise regularly. Always consult your doctor before you begin any exercise routine, but once that is done and you've been cleared, make a schedule. Use SheaNetics at least two or three times per week, and add in cardio that fits with your time and ability. Once you begin, you must show Perseverance, especially when your resolve is tested, as it most naturally will be in the early stages. Demonstrate Self-Control too by taking responsibility for your actions—no excuses. The more effort you invest in making good decisions, the easier it will be to sustain the effort and the sooner it will become a natural part of your lifestyle. Have the Integrity to try your best at all times. The body is more flexible and easier to work with on some days than on others. You should be forgiving of yourself when it's not easy, but always strive to set higher standards for yourself. By doing so you are showing Love, the care you have for yourself and your health, and setting a good example for others to follow.

You too can have a Breakthrough. Reading this book and learning how to apply The 5 Living Principles of Well-Being to your own life has already set you on the right road to wellness. In fact, understanding that you need or want a healthier lifestyle is a Breakthrough in and of itself! So you are already on your way, but in the next chapter I want to give your journey to well-being a big boost!

CHAPTER EIGHT

Shea's Five-Day Breakthrough Boost

Wellness is the journey and well-being
is the destination.

—Shea Vaughn

Wellness is a multidimensional concept that encourages you to bring health and balance into all aspects of your life—mind, body, and heart. The product of your achievement is a personal state of well-being. My five-day Breakthrough Boost is designed to be your first stop on the road to success in all that you do. Whether you are gearing up to infuse wellness into your life socially, financially, occupationally, physically, or emotionally, you can begin right now. Your body, mind, and heart must be engaged in the pursuit of Breakthroughs to promote wellness. The five-day Breakthrough Boost incorporates the practical and inspirational engines in this book, including The 5 Living Principles of Well-Being and the upcoming SheaNetics sequences to jump start your Breakthrough.

Wellness and Well-Being

The 5 Living Principles of Well-Being are the result of my personal study of the mental and emotional sides of exercise in order to understand my own motivation, and these have become the philosophical cornerstone of SheaNetics. They are meditation in thought. When the Principles are coupled with my unique exercises, SheaNetics becomes meditation in motion and thought—inspiring and guiding all you do and creating positive energy in your body, mind, and heart.

Many exercise programs are well-meaning, but without addressing the role of the mind and heart in finding wellness, they will only result in giving you short-term physical improvement. I want to reaffirm for you here how the Principles extend beyond just the physical to continuously drive beneficial Breakthroughs in all aspects of your life. SheaNetics is further unparalleled because it is based on the fact that the real goal for all of us is to find total health and fulfillment that lasts for life.

What better way to begin than to give you a system you can customize and try right now? For five days you can live the SheaNetics lifestyle—chock-full of affirmations that represent each Principle, a SheaNetics exercise sequence, and some of my favorite recipes that promote wellness and well-being—with the life-changing results for which SheaNetics is renowned.

Devote your attention to one Principle each day and "Embrace It, Own It, Live It®"—or try all five at once—and you will see changes in your outlook instantly. The best thing about the Boost is there is no right or wrong way to approach it. The Boost is yours to use in any fashion that works for you, and repetition will make it a natural part of your daily routine. Go ahead and reward yourself. Give your Breakthrough a Boost and discover SheaNetics as your pathway to well-being—starting now.

DAY ONE

Commitment

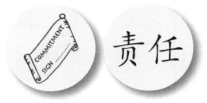

Breakthrough Behavior:

Visualize the power within you and unleash your greatness through Commitment.

Mind Boost:

- Set a realistic goal that is attainable.
- Be dedicated to your cause.
- Visualize yourself keeping the promise.
- Do not waver in the face of opposing viewpoints.
- Do not use fear as an excuse to second-guess yourself.
- For every commitment made to another, also make one to yourself.
- Consider all options before making a decision and then stand by it.
- Remember that each day is a new opportunity to make lasting changes.

- Just show up, and you are halfway closer to succeeding.
- Make you and your promise a priority.

Body Boost:

This standing sequence takes your body through multiple directions and causes you to commit your entire body to motion right from the start. As you perform each pose, you use strength to extend the stretch. This sequence is repeated on both sides of the body at least four times. Combine it with my smoothie recipe for a healthy way to jump-start your day with energy.

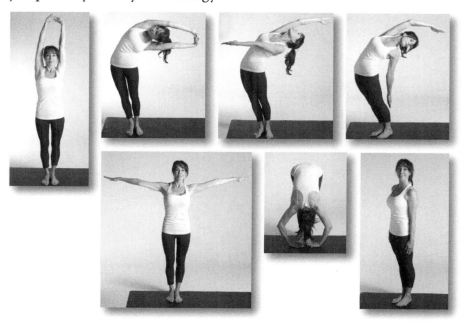

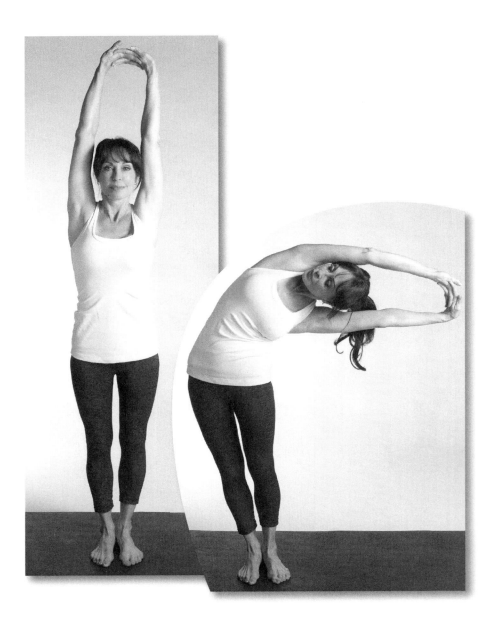

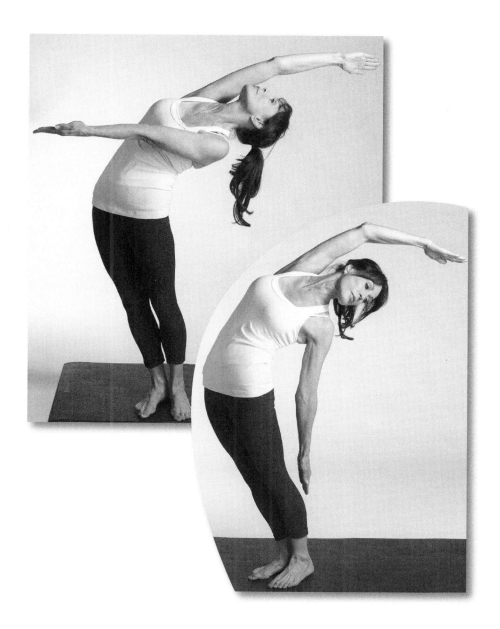

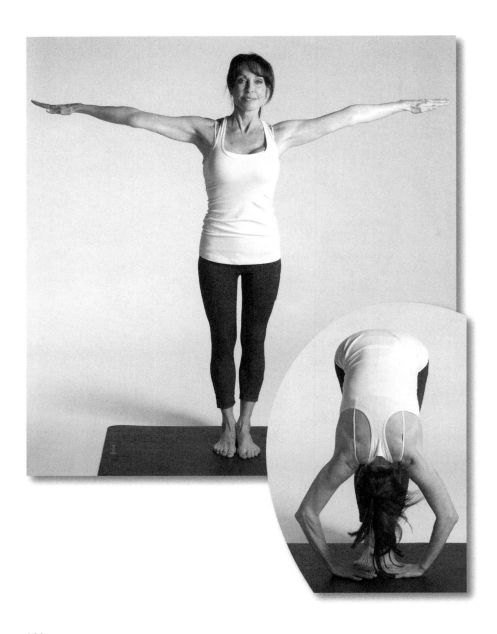

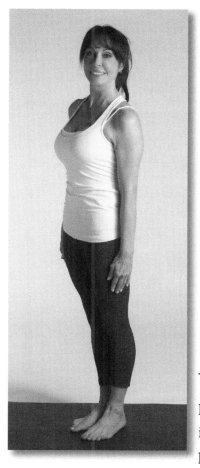

Nutrition Boost:

This smoothie recipe that follows is perfect for a grab-and-go snack or an ideal pick-me-up for the day. The cod liver oil is high in omega-3 fatty acids, which will help your mind to stay focused, and the protein and the greens provide you with substantial energy. You'll get an added boost of antioxidants from the blueberries and the apples. I always recommend organic produce whenever you can get it.

SHEA'S HEALTHY ENERGY SMOOTHIE

2 tbsps. Udo's Oil 3-6-9 Blend

2 tbsps. organic flaxseed oil *(high lignan)*

2 tbsps. Artic Cod Liver Oil

2 tbsps. liquid calcium magnesium

1 heaping tbsp. organic hemp protein powder
(chocolate or your choice of flavor)

1 scoop energy greens, Orac or Barleans *(scoop provided in container)*

2 generous tsps. cashew, almond, or
organic crunchy peanut butter

2 tbsps. blueberries *(or your choice of fruit)*

½ apple *(always include apples; they're high in
nutritional value and add flavor)*

½ cup almond or coconut milk

1 tsp. of raw agave nectar *(agave is a desert plant that
is sweet like a dessert)*

½ cup ice and ½ cup water
(add less or more to obtain your desired consistency when blended)

Blend all ingredients until they are completely mixed and the drink has a smooth consistency.

DAY TWO

Perseverance

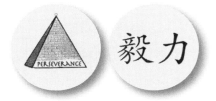

Breakthrough Behavior:

Call upon your willpower to heighten your focus and drive energy to its highest point.

Mind Boost:

- Stay focused on the task at hand.

- Nothing is worse than false starts—not even failure.

- Stay on course, even in the face of conflict.

- Think of losses as gains, as obstacles that hold the greatest learning experiences.

- Repetition is the key to reinforcing good behavior.

- Keep trying, no matter what—you owe it to yourself.

- Set milestones and review your progress.

- Let others know your goal; they will become your cheerleaders.

- Be disciplined, and when you waver, remind yourself of your promise.
- Just keep moving in the right direction: forward.

Body Boost:

This sequence is a combination of two SheaNetics moves called Tail Feather and Airplane. This and the following poses are challenging and require Perseverance. Remember, if you find it too difficult you can modify a move. However, try harder each time you repeat the sequence, because Breakthroughs come from sticking to it and aspiring to a higher level of performance each time.

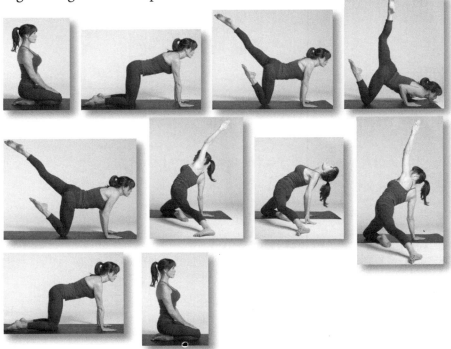

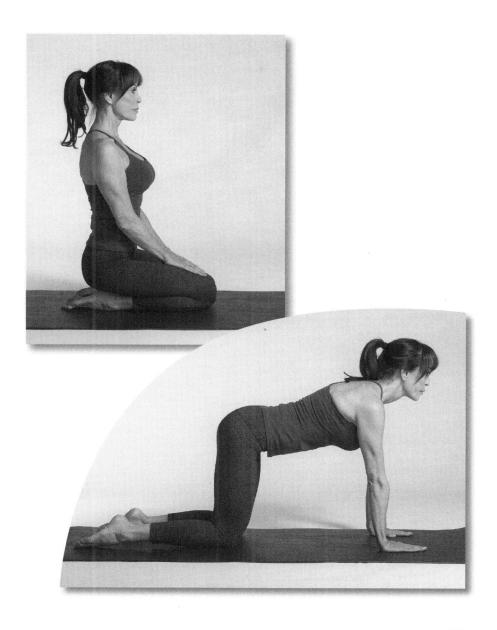

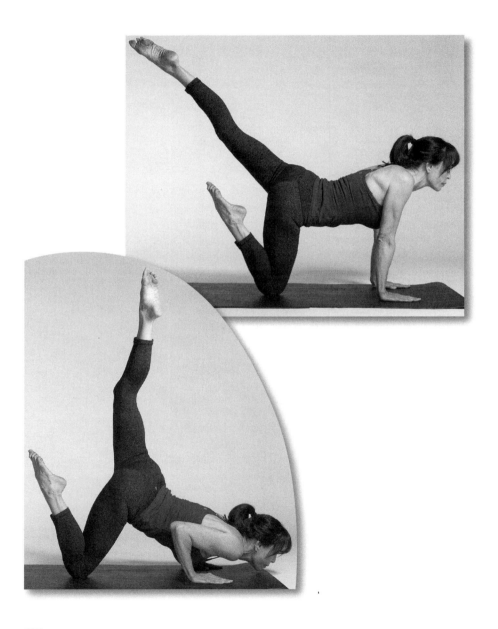

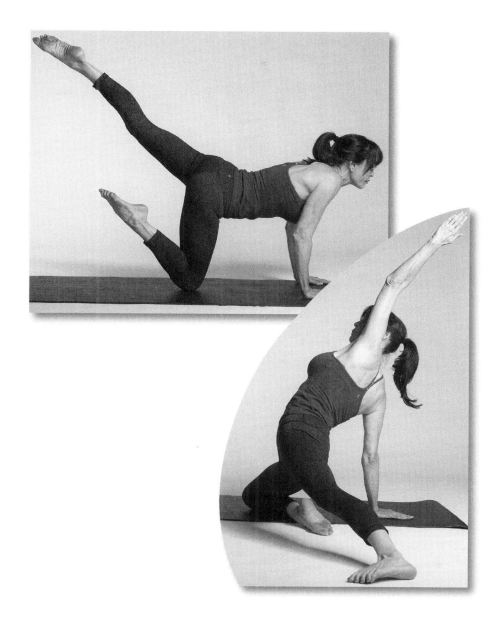

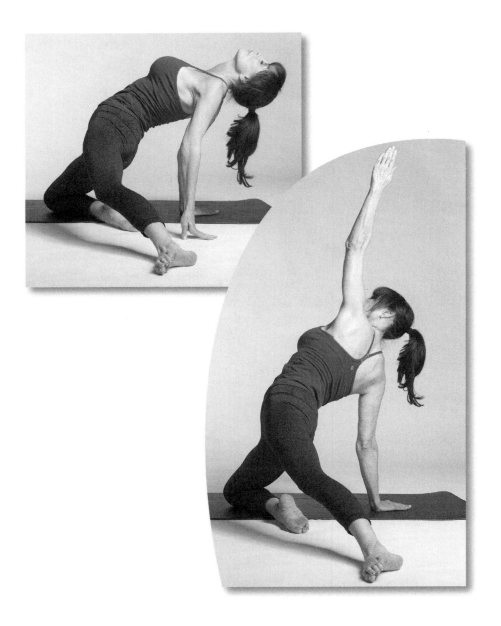

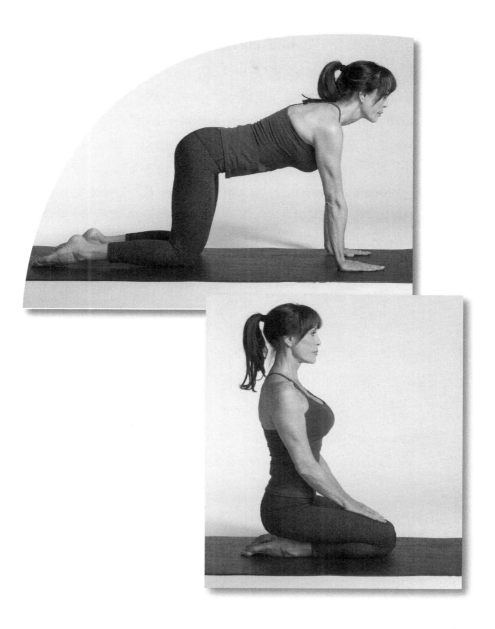

Nutrition Boost:

This lettuce wrap is easy and simple for a quick lunch or snack. You can follow the recipe or pick your favorite vegetables, and add meat if you desire. Bugs Bunny wasn't the only one that knew lettuce is full of calcium, iron, and vitamins C and K. The cucumber is 90 percent water and a great way to increase your fiber, and the tomato increases your nutritional intake with vitamins C, A, and B. A wrap doesn't get any better than this!

LETTUCE WRAP

1 large lettuce leaf, washed and dried

1 tbsp. hummus *(enough to coat the leaf or more, if desired)*

Tomato, 2 to 3 pieces thinly sliced

Cucumber, 4 pieces peeled and thinly sliced

Bell pepper, 2 to 3 pieces thinly sliced

Spread the hummus on the lettuce leaf and cover with the tomato, cucumber, and pepper slices. Use more ingredients if desired, and choose organic whenever possible. Salt and pepper to taste, if necessary, and then roll it up tightly. It's messy but delicious! For variety, add another vegetable such as spinach, or some meat such as chicken.

DAY THREE

Self-Control

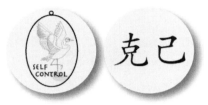

Breakthrough Behavior:

Be mindful and bring active awareness to every thought, move, and action. Calmness and balance will emerge.

Mind Boost:

- Do not allow negative thoughts to sabotage your endeavors.
- Practice restraint in the face of aggressive behavior.
- Do not project your insecurities onto those who criticize you.
- Greet your enemies with kindness and positive energy.
- Draw reasonable boundaries and be responsible for your behavior.
- Keep a level head. Do not get overwhelmed; work through it.
- Keep to the program and your routine.

- Take a deep breath when experiencing upsetting emotions.
- Tell yourself, "Patience is key in all things."
- Visualize yourself as calm and in control.

Body Boost:

Execution of this sequence requires complete focus and Self-Control in your mind and body. Set aside distractions, create a feedback loop between your mind and your body to calm yourself, and make minor adjustments to find and maintain your balance. Complement your equilibrium with cuisine choices that are equally harmonious.

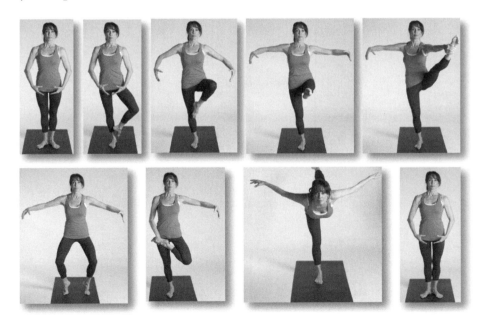

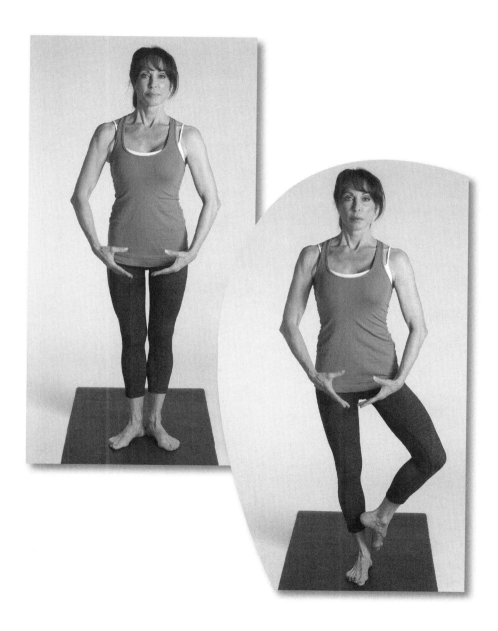

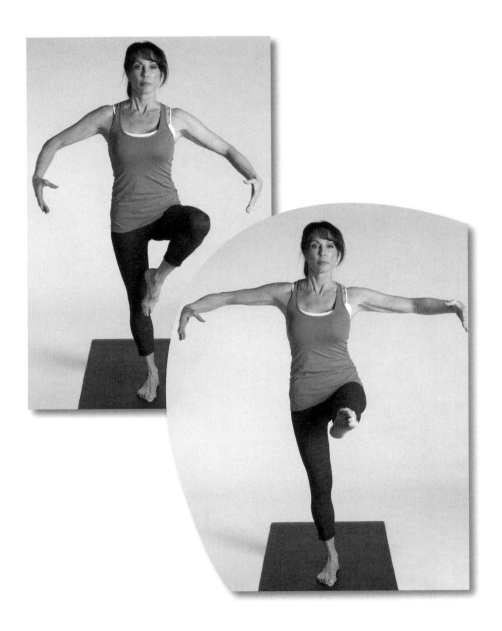

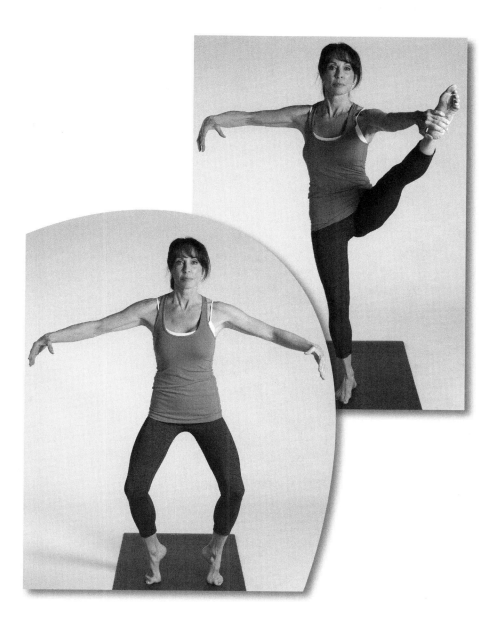

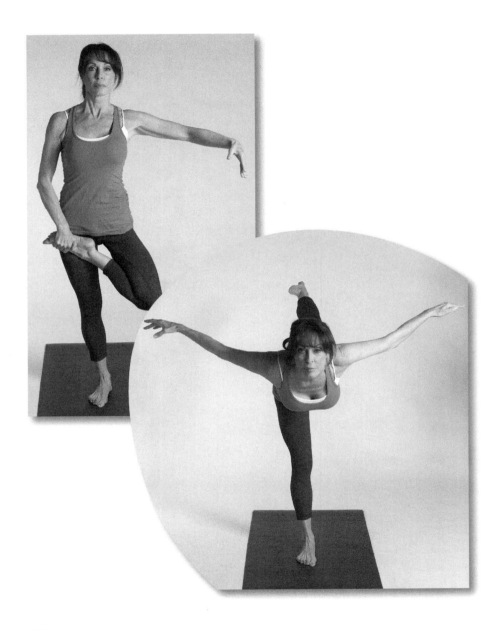

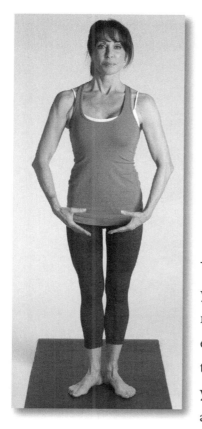

Nutrition Boost:

This meal will bring some balance to your menu. Lentil soup is a great-tasting meal any time of the day. Lentils are especially good for vegetarians because they are rich in protein. Onions, which you may not know, are cultivated in almost every country around the world. They provide our body with calcium, protein, vitamins A and C, and no fats. Garlic makes everything taste better and also has many nutritional benefits, including vitamins A, C, D, B1, B6, and B12. Salads can be packed full of valuable nutrients, depending on the variety of vegetables you put in them. Of course, the amount of calories in your salad will vary depending on whether you add cheese, nuts, or protein and the type of salad dressing you add, if any. I have to say salads are one of my "must-have" things to eat and enjoy. Fruits supply fresh vitamins, minerals, and enzymes. There is nothing better than cold fresh watermelon, especially when it is warm outside. We all should eat more fruit and leave the other desserts alone.

BALANCED DINNER:
SOUP, SALAD, AND DESSERT

Serves 4

LENTIL SOUP

1 tbsp. extra virgin olive oil

2 medium carrots, thinly sliced

4 celery stalks, thinly sliced

2 garlic cloves, minced

1 onion, diced

1½ cups lentils; rinse thoroughly and drain removing any small stones

1 cup water *(and possibly more)*

3 cups vegetable broth *(and possibly more)*

1 14-ounce can stewed tomatoes

½ tsp. salt

¼ tsp. black pepper

¼ tsp. ground cumin

¼ tsp. ground coriander

2 bay leaves

½ tsp. dry thyme

½ tsp. fresh parsley, chopped

Heat olive oil in a large saucepan over medium heat. Add carrots, celery, garlic, and onions and sauté for two minutes. Add lentils and then stir in the water, vegetable broth, and stewed tomatoes. Add the salt, pepper, thyme, coriander, and bay leaves. Bring to boil, reduce heat, and simmer for approximately 45 minutes or until the lentils are tender. Ladle the soup into warm bowls and garnish with parsley and serve. The soup can also be served over cooked brown rice or noodles. Add extra vegetable broth to obtain the liquid consistency you desire.

Salad

1½ cups spinach, washed

1½ cups mixed greens, washed

½ cucumber, peeled and sliced

1 tomato, diced

4 radishes, diced

2 medium oranges, peeled and diced
(save extra juice in a bowl)

⅓ cup chopped cashews
(or other nuts of your choice)

4 fresh dates, pitted and diced

Juice of ¼–½ lemon

Salt

Pepper

Assemble all the solid ingredients in a medium-sized bowl. For the dressing, mix the remaining orange juice, the lemon juice, and salt and pepper to taste. Shake well and pour over the salad just before serving.

Fresh Fruit Dessert

1 mango, peeled and diced

2 cups diced strawberries

1 banana, sliced

1 cup blueberries

1 cup raspberries

½ pineapple, diced

¼ cup fresh mint leaves, chopped fine

3 tablespoons honey, if desired

Place all of the fruit except the raspberries in a large bowl. Add the honey, if using, and stir gently until incorporated. Add the raspberries and mint and give the salad one final careful stir making sure that the raspberries don't get crushed. Serve immediately or chill in the refrigerator. The beauty of this salad is that it is not only healthy but very adaptable; experiment with your favorite fruits or any fruits that are in season, choosing organic whenever you can. The mint is a nice accompaniment and really makes the fruit flavors pop.

DAY FOUR

Integrity

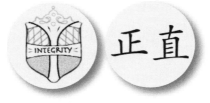

Breakthrough Behavior:

Approach your life with courage and be responsible for every outcome. With truth comes honor.

Mind Boost:

- Always act with good intentions.
- Do not compromise by cutting corners.
- Trust your instincts and act in accordance with your principles.
- Focus on the efforts made, not on the results.
- When your beliefs and standards are questioned, stand tall.
- Make a new start by addressing unfinished business.
- Be honest when you evaluate yourself.

- Do the right thing, even when no one is watching.

- Make a 100 percent effort to be the person you want to be.

- Always smile and put your best foot forward.

Body Boost:

This sequence calls on you to make each effort your best. Each pose and transition summons your Tri-Core Power and challenges you to execute every move with honest conviction.

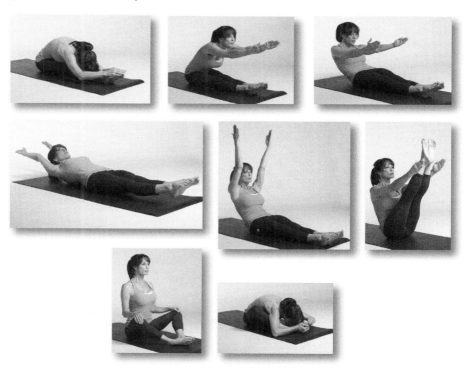

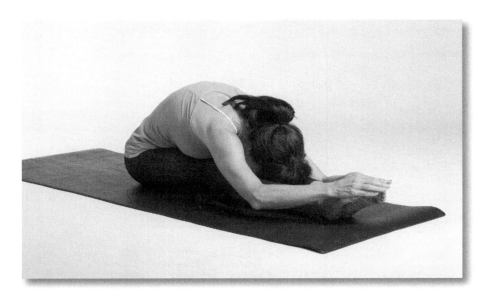

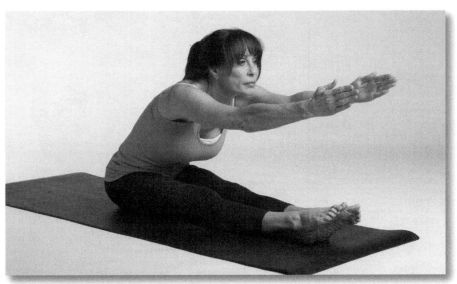

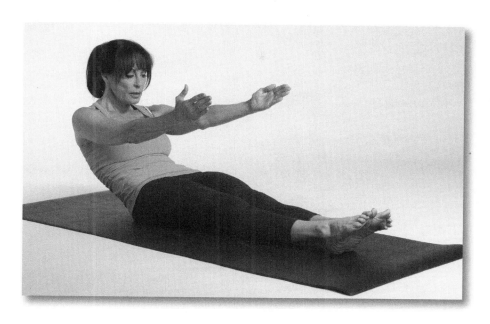

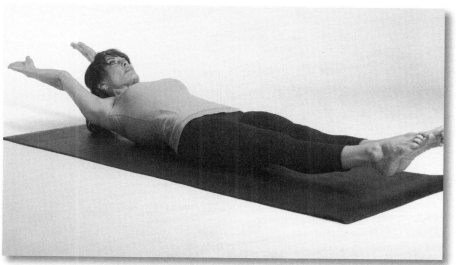

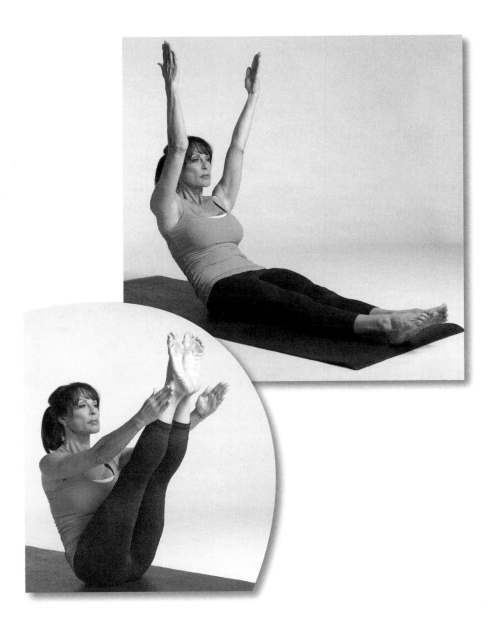

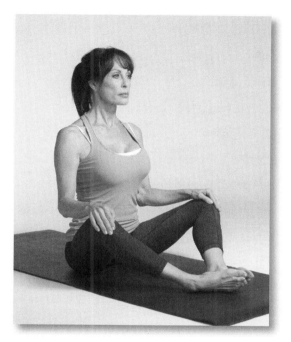

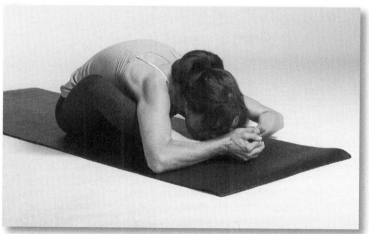

Nutrition Boost:

I love dips, and especially this one because it is so quick and easy to make and is packed with nutritional benefits. Olive oil is used throughout the world, but especially in Mediterranean cooking. Olive oil is an antioxidant and, if you consume it regularly, it can help modulate your blood pressure. Onions are fat-free and provide vitamins A and C, calcium, and protein, and the beans are a good source of vitamin B6. If you are skeptical about vegan products, don't be: the Daiya vegan cheese shreds, melts, and tastes delicious. If you have company over and serve this dip, it will make a huge hit.

EASY BEAN DIP

1 tbsp. extra virgin olive oil

1 medium onion, chopped

1 15-oz. can organic refried beans

4 oz. organic salsa

1 cup Daiya vegan cheese-style shreds

1 15-oz. can organic pinto beans

Heat olive oil in a skillet and sauté onions until translucent. Reduce heat and add all other ingredients. Cook over low heat until shreds melt and blend.

Serve with rice, crackers, and bite-sized pieces of veggies.

DAY FIVE

Love

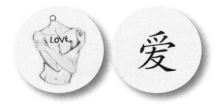

Breakthrough Behavior:

Connect to each heart with the gift of support, then your intentions and actions will contribute purposefully to the greater well-being of all.

Mind Boost:

- Give yourself permission to love yourself.
- Forgive yourself for yesterday's mistakes and move on.
- Find time to nurture yourself as you nurture those you love.
- Put yourself in other people's shoes; try to consider their points of view and do not judge.
- Think in terms of setting the best example by your actions.
- Be grateful to others for the things they do, big and small, without keeping track.
- Congratulate yourself for making better choices.

- Embrace what you can do and be forgiving for what you find challenging.
- Allow others to be strong.
- Hug and love yourself.

Body Boost:

The Love you possess and wish to share with others resonates from this sequence. The graceful moves express the inner beauty that is the essence of your being and further reflects an instinctive call to connect with others. Love is universal.

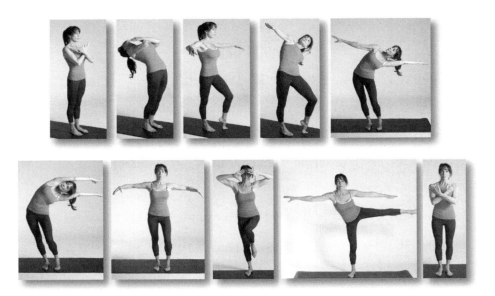

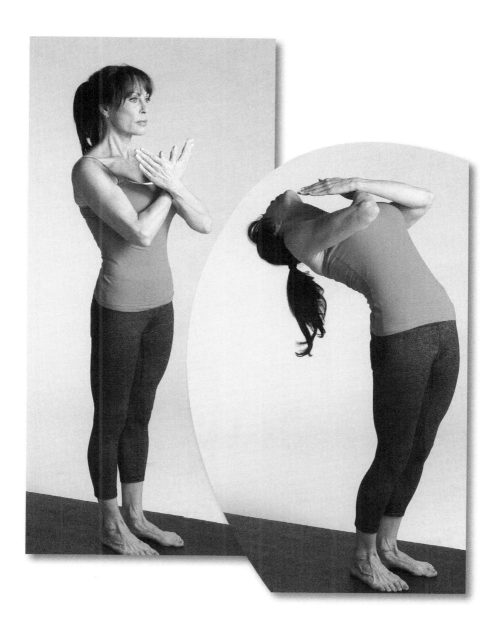

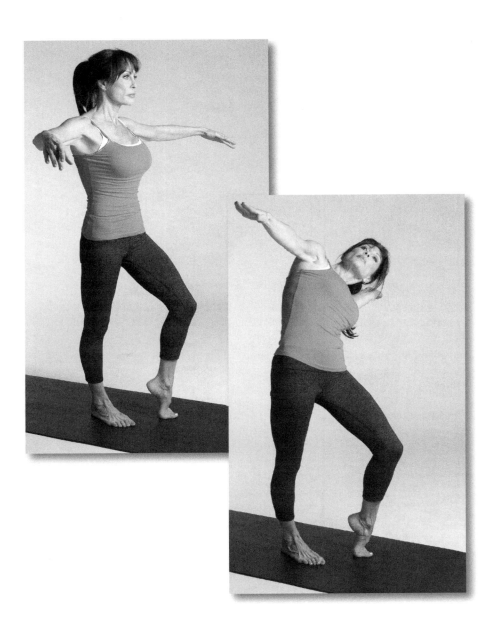

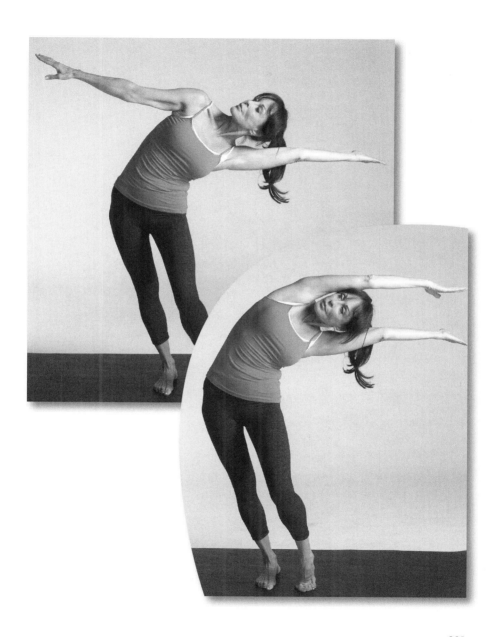

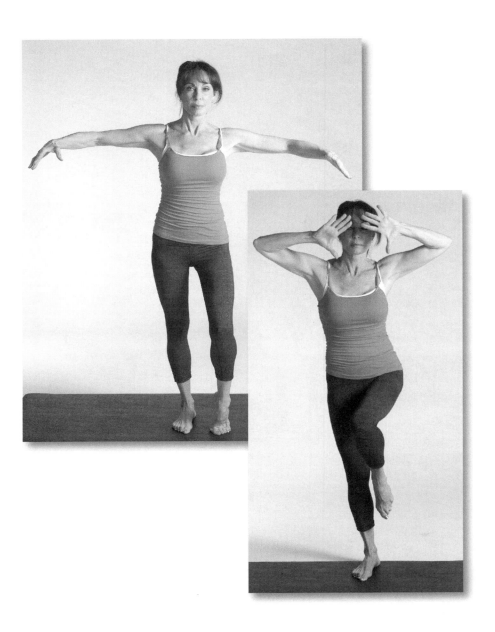

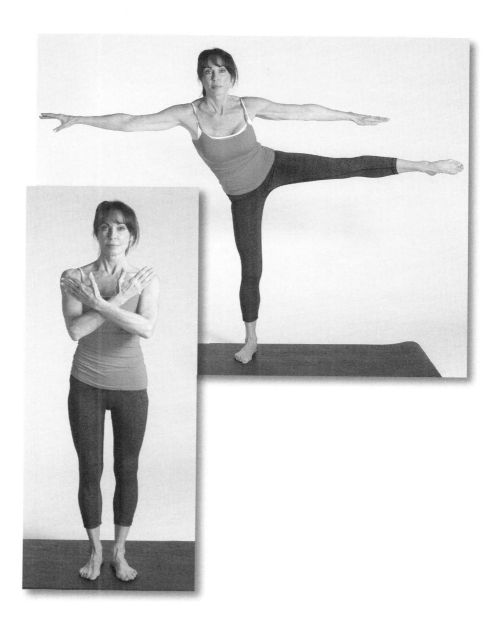

Nutrition Boost:

I love hummus and sweet, red grapes are my favorite for dipping. I can make a meal out of just this! Hummus provides protein, iron, and manganese, and there are many flavorful varieties of grapes that are high in nutritional value with vitamins A and C and other minerals. I also like to chill the grapes in the refrigerator and make a refreshing snack for on-the-go. But you can add any raw vegetable or even apples to the dip, if you prefer.

HUMMUS RECIPE

2½ cups garbanzo beans *(chickpeas)*

3 garlic cloves

⅔ cup tahini

1 tsp. salt

Juice squeezed from ½ of a large lemon

2 tbsps. extra virgin olive oil

Paprika to garnish

I prefer to use large dried beans. Soak them overnight and then rinse and cook to desired tenderness (also see package instructions). Place all ingredients except olive oil in blender and mix until desired texture. Scoop into a bowl and drizzle 2 tbsps. of olive oil over the top and sprinkle lightly with paprika.

New Beginnings

These may be the last pages of the book, but it is not the end; I believe it is the beginning. I hope you have felt like you were sitting comfortably, chatting with your best friend, who in return provided you with loving and positive options to help you on your continued journey to a state of well-being. The 5 Living Principles of Well-Being are transforming and will continue to be your life companion. They will always, without fail, help you with every decision, every encounter, and whatever life puts in your way.

Breakthroughs are the perfect blend of clarity, wisdom, and truth. As you open your heart to the possibilities, you move forward with enlightenment. Life has joined us together with no significant differences. Each of us seeks self-meaning and purpose. Your road map may take you on an alternate route, but ultimately we all travel to a common destination, where we hope to find harmony, peace, balance, and love.

This is a time of opportunity to explore yourself and the impact you have on others by taking advantage of the insight you experience through your Breakthrough. Knowledge gives us freedom to firmly plant our feet in tomorrow's dreams as well as confidence to make our dreams our reality. I hope the view you have of yourself and the way you choose to live your life will forever be your greatest Breakthrough, leaving all regrets behind and being grateful every morning when the sun comes up.

I hope the view you have of yourself and the way you choose to live your life will forever be your greatest Breakthrough.

About Shea Vaughn

Shea Vaughn is a fitness expert, professional trainer, and wellness coach with a lifetime of mind-body experience and a passion for health and well-being. She has gained national recognition as an inspirational speaker and media personality and is admired by a devoted group of students and clients, including athletes and celebrities—helping them all to build strength and flexibility, prevent injuries, "stay in the game" and live more fulfilling lives.

Shea is the CEO and founder of SheaNetics®, a revolutionary lifestyle, wellness, and exercise practice that blends Eastern and Western values and movements for a powerful mind-body experience. You get in shape, feel great, and naturally make healthy choices.

The heart of SheaNetics is The 5 Living Principles of Well-Being—Commitment, Perseverance, Self-Control, Integrity, and Love; uniting the mind and body as one and inspiring the answers you seek—to live the life you want. SheaNetics takes mind-body transformation one step further with a fresh self-styled approach to exercise that combines yoga, pilates, tai chi, martial arts, ballet, and lots more, along with the performance-enhancing benefits of *Tri-Core Power Training*—to develop your "killer" core. SheaNetics is "Your Pathway to Well-Being."

Shea began her career in health and wellness as a dancer and teacher and later broadened her scope as a fitness instructor and trainer with an impressive resume of program and specialist certifications. She has recently released the SheaNetics 6-Disc DVD/CD Mind-Body collection and has been a featured guest with Lululemon Apparel, The Home Shopping Group, and QVC. Go to *www.sheanetics.com*.

Index